Heart Failure

Strategies to Improve Outcomes

The Cardiovascular Team Approach

A book series focusing on the interprofessional team approach for the management and prevention of cardiovascular diseases.

Look for these and other forthcoming series titles from Cardiotext Publishing.

Volume 1: *Heart Failure: Strategies to Improve Outcomes*
Ileana L. Piña, MD, MPH, FACC, FAHA, and
Elizabeth A. Madigan, PhD, RN, FAAN, editors

Volume 2: *Prehospital Management of the Acute Infarction Patient*
Edgardo Escobar, MD, FACC, FAHA, and
Alejandro Barbagelata, MD, FAHA, FSCAI, editors

Volume 3: *Acute Coronary Syndrome: Urgent and Follow-up Care*
Eileen Handberg, PhD, ARNP, BC, FAHA, FACC, and
R. David Anderson, MD, MS, FACC, FSCAI, editors

Please visit www.cardiotextpublishing.com for more information about this series.

Heart Failure

Strategies to Improve Outcomes

The Cardiovascular Team Approach

Ileana L. Piña, MD, MPH, FACC, FAHA
Elizabeth A. Madigan, PhD, RN, FAAN
Volume Editors

Joseph S. Alpert, MD, FAHA, FACC, MACP, FESC
Lynne T. Braun, PhD, CNP, FAHA, FAAN
Barbara J. Fletcher, RN, MN, FAHA, FAAN
Gerald Fletcher, MD, FAHA
Editors-in-chief

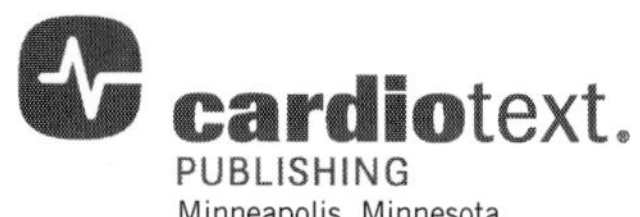

Cardiotext Publishing, LLC
3405 W. 44th Street
Minneapolis, Minnesota 55410
USA

www.cardiotextpublishing.com

Any updates to this book may be found at: www.cardiotextpublishing.com/titles/detail/9781935395508

Comments, inquiries, and requests for bulk sales can be directed to the publisher at: info@cardiotextpublishing.com

Library of Congress Control Number: 2013931846

ISBN: 978-1-935395-50-8

Printed in the United States of America.

Dedicated to my daughter, Victoria, who continues to be my inspiration and garners my admiration for her integrity and incredible strength.

—Ileana L. Piña

I wish to acknowledge the support of my husband, Glenn, and children, Tom and Leigh, and the many patients with heart failure I have cared for during my career.

—Elizabeth A. Madigan

Contents

About the Editors-in-chief

Editors-in-chief

Joseph S. Alpert, MD, FAHA, FACC, MACP, FESC
Professor of Medicine
University of Arizona Health Science Network
Editor-in-chief, *The American Journal of Medicine*
Tucson, Arizona

Lynne T. Braun, PhD, CNP, FAHA, FAAN
Professor
Department of Adult Health and Gerontological Nursing
Rush University College of Nursing
Nurse Practitioner
Section of Cardiology, Rush University Medical Center
Chicago, Illinois

Barbara J. Fletcher, RN, MN, FAHA, FAAN
Clinical Associate Professor
Brooks College of Health, School of Nursing
University of North Florida
Jacksonville, Florida

Gerald Fletcher, MD, FAHA
Professor in Medicine (Cardiovascular Diseases)
Mayo Clinic College of Medicine
Mayo Clinic Florida
Jacksonville, Florida

About the Authors

Editors

Ileana L. Piña, MD, MPH, FACC, FAHA
Professor, Department of Medicine and Department of Epidemiology and Population Health
Associate Chief for Academic Affairs
Division of Cardiology
Staff Heart Failure/Transplant
Montefiore Einstein Center for Heart and Vascular Care
Bronx, New York

Elizabeth A. Madigan, PhD, RN, FAAN
Professor of Nursing
Frances Payne Bolton School of Nursing
Case Western Reserve University
Cleveland, Ohio

Contributors

Nancy Altice, DNP, RN, CCNS, ACNS-BC
Cardiology Clinical Nurse Specialist
Carilion Roanoke Memorial Hospital
Roanoke, Virginia

Angela Cheng-Lai, PharmD, BCPS
Clinical Pharmacy Manager
Montefiore Einstein Medical Center
Assistant Professor of Medicine
Department of Pharmacy
Albert Einstein College of Medicine
Bronx, New York

Miriam Pappo, MS, RD, CDN
Director, Clinical Nutrition
Montefiore Medical Center
Bronx, New York

Snehal Patel, MD
Department of Cardiology, Center for Advanced Cardiac Therapy
Montefiore Einstein Center for Heart and Vascular Care
Bronx, New York

Xiomara Tolentino, LMSW
Social Worker/Discharge Planner
Montefiore Qualified Medical Interpreter
Montefiore Einstein Medical Center
Social Services Department
Bronx, New York

Preface

Heart failure is a complex syndrome. The approach to heart failure is equally complex. It is naïve to believe that one clinician can provide such needed complex care that is multifaceted and addresses not only the multiplicity of etiologies of heart failure but involves family and caregiver; provides ongoing education, support, and nutritional advice; and takes into consideration the psychosocial aspects of each patient. It is, in fact, impossible. This book presents the true multidisciplinary approach to this common syndrome. The authors are professionals who actively practice and care for heart failure patients, each in their own specialty. The book is not meant to be a cookbook for care but a guide that opens doors to the possibilities.

Ileana L. Piña

Abbreviations

ACC	American College of Cardiology
ACE	angiotensin-converting enzyme
ACEI	ACE inhibitor
ADA	American Diabetes Association
ADHERE	Acute Decompensated Heart Failure Registry
AHA	American Heart Association
AII	angiotensin II
APRN	advanced practice registered nurse
ARB	angiotensin II receptor blocker
AV	arteriovenous
BMI	body mass index
BNP	brain natriuretic peptide
CAD	coronary artery disease
CBC	complete blood count
CES-D	Center for Epidemiologic Studies–Depression
COPD	chronic obstructive pulmonary disease
CRT	cardiac resynchronization therapy
CVD	cardiovascular disease
EF	ejection fraction
EFI	executive function impairment
FDA	U.S. Food and Drug Administration
GFR	glomerular filtration rate
HEENT	head, eyes, ears, nose, and throat
HF	heart failure
HF-ACTION	Heart Failure: A Controlled Trial Investigating Outcomes of Exercise Training
HFpEF	heart failure with preserved ejection fraction
HFREF	heart failure with reduced ejection fraction
HMO	health maintenance organization

H2H	American College of Cardiology Hospital to Home program
ICD	implantable cardioverter–defibrillator
JVP	jugular venous pressure
LBBB	left bundle branch block
LIP	licensed independent provider
LV	left ventricular
LVEF	left ventricular ejection fraction
MERIT-HF	Metoprolol CR/XL Randomized Intervention Trial in Congestive Heart Failure
MI	myocardial infarction
MMSE	Mini Mental Status Exam
MNT	medical nutrition therapy
NP	nurse practitioner
n-3 PUFA	n-3 polyunsaturated fatty acids
NYHA	New York Heart Association
PA	physician assistant
PAI-1	plasminogen activator inhibitor-1
PHQ2	Patient Health Questionnaire-2
RAAS	renin-angiotensin-aldosterone system
RCT	randomized controlled trial
RD	registered dietitian
RN	registered nurse
RV	right ventricular
SNS	sympathetic nervous system
SOB	shortness of breath
SOLVD	Studies of Left Ventricular Dysfunction
URI	upper respiratory infection
VA	U.S. Department of Veterans Affairs
VAD	ventricular assist device

Introduction

THE INTEGRATED TEAM APPROACH TO THE CARE OF THE PATIENT WITH CARDIOVASCULAR DISEASE

Authors: Gerald Fletcher, MD[1], Kathy Berra, MSN, NP[2], Barbara J. Fletcher, RN, MN[3], Lauren Gilstrap, MD[4], Malissa J. Wood, MD[5]

Affiliations: [1]Department of Cardiovascular Diseases at Mayo Clinic, Jacksonville, FL; [2]Stanford Prevention Research Center, Stanford University, Palo Alto, CA; [3]School of Nursing, Brooks College of Health, University of North Florida, Jacksonville, FL; [4]Resident in Internal Medicine, Massachusetts General Hospital, Boston, MA; [5]Cardiovascular Diseases, Massachusetts General Hospital, Boston, MA

The management of cardiovascular disease (CVD) requires intensive and sustained efforts to effectively prevent death, disability, and substantial personal and societal costs. Research reveals that a comprehensive and team-based approach to primary and secondary prevention is critical to achieve a reduction in the incidence of CVD and in the recovery from an acute CVD event. Not only is this a responsibility of the healthcare professional and the patients at risk, families and communities are also involved. Families have been shown to play a critical role in the prevention of chronic illness in children and adults. Families with healthy lifestyles predict healthy

Reprinted from Current Problems in Cardiology, September 2012, 2012;37:369-397, with permission from Elsevier.

adult lifestyle habits and improved CVD risk factors.[1-3] Thus, the care of persons with and at risk for CVD has evolved to emcompass complex management strategies far beyond the one-doctor-one-patient model of care.

Historical Perspective of Team-based Care

The team approach in the management of the patients with CVD has its roots in a pattern of care that evolved many years ago.[4] Early physicians are often pictured with a nurse or a family member acting as an assistant. This practice was considered essential in the care of the patient, be it in the home, office, or infirmary. This partnership in care provided a more comprehensive management strategy when compared to the physician alone. This comprehensive care was manifested in the development and use of surgical instruments, preparation of and administering of medications, and counseling and comforting of the patient. Certainly this is true today in our multiple-member teams, albeit in a more sophisticated and organized manner. As medical education, training, and medical schools evolved, medical and nursing students and trainees “made rounds” as a team with physicians as they cared for their patients. Though the physician made the medical care decisions, the didactic interchange with the students likely influenced and improved patient care. One of the earlier and most successful team approaches evolved with the advent of the cardiac rehabilitation programs in the 1960s and 1970s. These programs developed on both national and international levels. On the national level, programs like Cleveland, Ohio; Atlanta, Georgia; Rochester, Minnesota; New York, New York; Seattle, Washington; and Palo Alto, California were the leaders. Internationally, programs in Germany, Finland, Sweden, Denmark, and France were well-known as pioneers in this area. These programs utilized a team approach to the care of patients with CVD. These team members included, but were not limited to:

- Physicians
- Nurses and advanced practice nurses
- Physical therapists
- Occupational therapists
- Exercise physiologists
- Dietitians
- Pharmacists
- Chaplains and spiritual counselors
- Recreational therapists

In this context, some of the original scientific clinical research was published relative to the team approach, especially with regard to the role of exercise in the patient with CVD.[5-11] Over time, the team concept has evolved in other subsets of care for the patient with CVD. In the discussion to follow, details will be presented and evidence will be provided to clarify and support the value of the integrated team in the care of the patient with CVD. In addition, methodology for the team-based approach will be clarified, and examples of successful integrated team approaches will be provided.

Integrated Team-based Care—What Is the Evidence?

Significant research has revealed that a collaborative care model is essential in the improved management of complex medical problems, including cardiovascular disease (Figure 1).[12-14] Collaborative care, team-based care, case/care managers, and systematic care all are team-based approaches in today's health-care system. Team-based care has shown great promise for hospitalized patients as well as outpatient management.

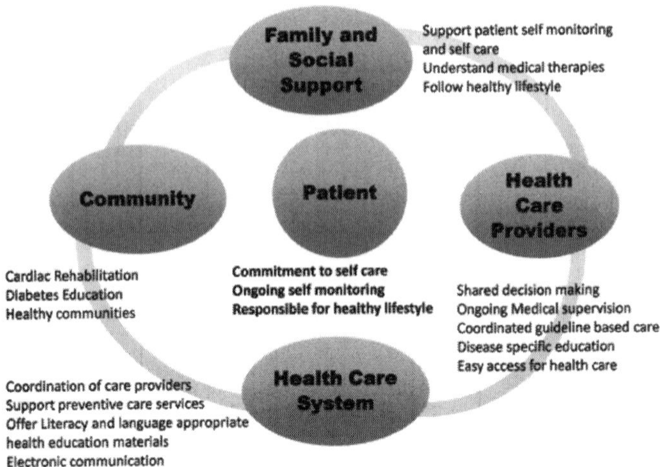

Figure 1

Team-based Care Model: Team-based care management represents selected responsibilities of the healthcare team including the patient, family and social support, healthcare providers, community, and the healthcare system. Specific responsibilities are listed by each component in this team-based care management illustration.

Significant work demonstrating the effectiveness of team-based care for patients with coronary artery disease has guided the implementation of such care into mainstream medicine. The MULTIFIT program revealed that, in patients following an acute myocardial infarction, guideline-based care implemented by a team of doctors, nurses, and nutritionists improved smoking cessation and cholesterol levels when compared to typical care.[15] The Stanford Coronary Risk Intervention Program demonstrated in men and women with documented coronary artery disease that a team of physicians, nurses, nutritionists, and psychologists were able to reduce angiographically measured atherosclerosis, total cardiovascular events, cardiovascular risk factors, and primary cardiac events in treated subjects versus control subjects.[16] Based on these studies and the many others that followed, EUROACTION was undertaken to evaluate the effectiveness of a team-based approach in the management of cardiovascular risk reduction in a variety of settings including hospital-based clinics and primary care or general practice settings. They demonstrate the benefits of a team of physicians, nurses, and dietitians in improving cardiovascular risk factors in the intervention group versus the control group.[17]

Nurse-based case management studies have shown that individualized, systematic, and guideline-based care results in the reduction of cardiovascular-related morbidity and mortality. These team-based approaches to improving care were shown to be effective for hospitalized patients, primary care patients, low-income clinics, in the workplace, and in community centers.[18] They demonstrated reduced mortality, recurrent myocardial infarction, and hospitalizations in the treatment group versus typical care. This was attributed to the success of the team to achieve guideline-based recommendations for CVD risk reduction and adherence to recommended medical therapies for myocardial infarction patients.[19]

Managing Cardiovascular Disease with an Integrated Approach

The management of CVD and other chronic conditions is a challenge for the healthcare system, patients, their families, providers, and society as a whole. Significant research and clinical programs have targeted the management of chronic illnesses by designing both efficient and cost-effective interventions.[20]

In one qualitative investigation, older persons were interviewed regarding specific needs they had in order to successfully manage their health conditions. All of the participants were members of a health maintenance organization (HMO). The respondents reported that their daily routines were greatly affected by their medical conditions, including their physical abilities, social support, self-management tasks, assessment of symptoms, and personal treatment decisions. In addition to their own healthcare needs, some of the respondents also had responsibilities for the care of a spouse and/or others. The main themes and concerns expressed were:

- Convenient access to providers
- Continuity of care
- Clear communication of the care plan
- Individualized and coordinated care
- Being "heard"[20]

Addressing these needs is multifactorial. It involves participation by the healthcare system, individual and group providers, patients, patients' families, and communities.

Models of comprehensive care for older persons with multiple comorbidities have been evaluated.[21] In a report by Boult et al., 15 positive studies were carefully analyzed and included in the final analysis. All of these studies reported improved outcomes in one or more of the following domains: quality of care, health outcomes, and efficiency. Ten of these models are listed in Table 1. Boult's analysis included results from healthcare models that supplemented primary care and provided transitional and acute care in patients' homes. In addition, they evaluated models of comprehensive care in hospitals and nurse-physician teams for nursing home residents. This report highlights the growing efficacy and efficiency of team-based models to improve healthcare delivery and, ultimately, healthcare outcomes.[21]

The role of the team in the implementation of guideline-based cardiovascular disease risk factor management has also been well studied and has shown to be beneficial. This finding

Table 1
Examples of Integrated Team-based Care Models with Key Outcomes[21]

Integrated Team-based Care Model	Key Outcomes
Care or Case Management	Better satisfaction with care, quality of care, quality of life, and survival
Interdisciplinary Primary Care	Reduce healthcare cost, reduce use of health services, increase survival
Outpatient Comprehensive Geriatric Assessment and Geriatric Evaluation and Management	Increase survival
Disease Management	Reduce use of health services
Chronic Disease Self-Management	Improve quality of life and functional autonomy
Proactive Rehabilitation	Potential for beneficial effects on physical function
Caregiver Education and Support	Reduce use of health services, improve quality of life and functional autonomy
Transitional Care	Reduce healthcare cost, improve quality of life and functional autonomy
Comprehensive Inpatient Care	Improve quality of life and functional autonomy
Early Discharge Hospital-to-Home	Improve patients' quality of life, reduce hospital utilization and healthcare costs

holds true worldwide and in the United States.[18] In a recent review of clinical trials addressing the achievement of guideline-based care for persons with CVD, important barriers and facilitators to the implementation of effective case management were noted. With nurse-led case/care management serving as the foundation of an effective team-based approach, understanding and addressing these barriers remains a major challenge to patients and clinicians. Key barriers include:

- Cost to the patient
- Lack of social support
- Provision of educational materials in the appropriate language and at appropriate literacy levels
- Flexibility in scheduling
- Easy access to the case manager[18]

It is imperative that healthcare providers continue to research and implement efficient and cost-effective team-based care. This type of care has been shown to improve quality of life and reduce morbidity and mortality. Creating systematic approaches to care holds promise to make these services cost-effective for individual patients and society.

Clinical Models of Team-based Care

Health Maintenance Organizations

Beginning with the MULTIFIT study in the 1990s through current population studies, the Kaiser HMO model of care has evaluated and implemented successful coordinated, multidisciplinary care.[15] Care for chronic kidney disease was evaluated in a large non-profit HMO versus referral to nephrology for persons with Stage 3 kidney disease. The HMO model provided coordinated care delivered by a team comprised of a nephrologist, pharmacy specialist, diabetes educator, dietitian, social worker, and nephrology nurse. Patients were eligible if they had Stage 3 kidney disease plus one or more additional chronic diseases such as hypertension or Type 2 diabetes. The team-based care included education, medication management, nephrology consultation, and management of metabolic abnormalities. Care plans were renegotiated and individualized at each team visit. After two years of follow-up, patients receiving team-based care demonstrated a slower decline in glomerular filtration rate when compared to traditional nephrology care.[20]

Another randomized trial (TEAMcare) included 14 primary care clinics for patients with complex medical conditions including diabetes, coronary heart disease (CHD), and depression. The TEAMcare approach added a nurse care coordinator to provide patient self-management skills, systematic follow-up, and improvement of care continuity with the primary care physicians. This systematic approach in a large HMO resulted in improved control of diabetes, depression, and coronary heart disease.[22]

The addition of guided care teams for older persons was evaluated regarding their use of health services. The nurse and primary care physician team provided:

- Comprehensive assessment
- Evidence-based care planning
- Monthly monitoring of symptoms and adherence to care plans
- Transitional care
- Coordination of healthcare professionals
- Support for self-management
- Support for family caregivers
- Enhanced access to community services

The addition of these important support and clinical services showed a significant reduction in home healthcare utilization. Other outcomes, such as use of emergency rooms, skilled nursing facilities, or primary care and specialty physician services, did not demonstrate statistical differences. The authors recommended continued research to better determine high-quality and cost-effective care. Of the HMO organizations involved in this study, the Kaiser HMO was the most successful, prompting the authors to emphasize Kaiser's "well-established culture that promotes and rewards team care, prevention, and avoidance of unnecessary care."[23]

The Ochsner Clinic

At Ochsner Clinic, the featured and most successful integrated team model is the Ventricular Assist Device Program. This team has a physician leader for overall program management. The multidisciplinary team includes:

- Nurses
- Device coordinators
- Social services
- Financial coordinators
- Physical therapy
- Dietitians
- Administrative support

Routine patient care/selection meetings are held biweekly. The team presents the patient findings, and the medical decision to implant the device is considered by all. During this process, team education is of paramount importance. Equipment education includes the function and purpose of the device and clarification of troubleshooting techniques. Patient care issues and discharge preparation are discussed in detail in these meetings.

The team approach is continued in the ambulatory/outpatient setting. The physician specialist in heart failure and the device coordinator have biweekly clinics with ongoing multidisciplinary assessment and documentation. There is close collaboration with the outpatient Coumadin clinic and with referring physicians (Hector Ventura, MD, FACC, FACP, personal communication, December 2011).

The Veterans Affairs

The United States Department of Veterans Affairs (VA) is charged with providing services to active duty military personnel, veterans, their dependants, and surviving spouses/children.[24] The VA system is divided into three sections: Veteran Benefits Administration, Veterans Health Administration, and

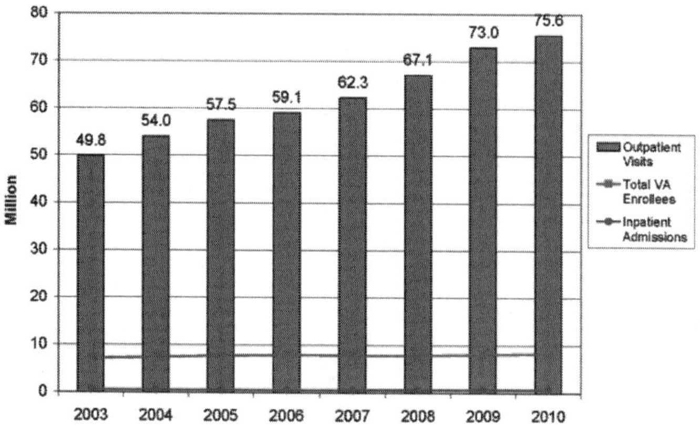

Figure 2

Utilization of Outpatient VA Care: While total VA enrollees and inpatient admissions for the system have remained flat over the past several years, outpatient visits have increased year by year. This increase in outpatient visits can be best facilitated by an integrated team approach.

the National Cemetery Administration. The Veterans Health Administration is responsible for all medical services provided by the VA system. In 2011, it comprised 152 medical centers, nearly 1,400 community-based outpatient clinics, community living centers, Vet Centers, and Domiciliaries.[25] In total, the Veterans Health Administration encompasses more than 53,000 independently licensed healthcare practitioners who provide care to approximately 8.3 million veterans each year (Figure 2).[26]

The VA is organized into 21 Veterans Integrated Service Networks, which are regional healthcare systems providing integrated primary care, specialty care, rehabilitation, mental health, and pharmacy services to geographic regions. In 2010, the VA spent approximately $108 billion—39%, or $42 billion, of which was for medical care. This covered 75.6 million outpatient clinic visits and 680,000 inpatient admissions.[26]

In addition to the population it serves, one of the other distinguishing attributes of the VA system is VistA—a system of approximately 100 integrated software modules built around the electronic medical record. VistA supports both ambulatory and inpatient care. It includes computerized order entry, bar code medication administration, e-prescribing, and clinical guideline reference. The most important feature for clinicians is the graphical user interface, Computerized Patient Record System.[27] The VistA electronic healthcare record has been credited for reforming the VA healthcare system and significantly improving both efficiency and safety.

Despite this, there is very little in the way of coordinated, team-based care. For inpatient service, every team has a Nurse Practitioner (NP), Advanced Practice Registered Nurse (APRN), or Physician Assistant (PA) to help coordinate care, in addition to the attending physician, fellow, resident, and intern. When it is determined that the patient requires ancillary services (nutrition, physical therapy, etc.), the cardiologist, APRN, or NP will request the consult, but there is no interdisciplinary team meeting. The consultant writes a formal consult note in the patient's record, and the primary team is responsible for determining what recommendations to implement.

For outpatients, there are additional services available though the VA, such as telemedicine and home-based follow-up visits. However, for general/preventive cardiology, there are no interdisciplinary teams or clinics. While there is no coordinated team-based care approach, individual attending physicians are beginning to create cardiology care teams. For example, over the past year, within the Heart Failure Clinic of the Boston VA system, an attending physician self-created a Heart Failure team, which follows heart failure patients in the outpatient setting. The team is composed of the cardiac fellows, APRNs, and NPs that care for the patient, but does not include interdisciplinary resources such as nutrition or physical therapy. There have been efforts to integrate the VA cardiology clinic with the nearby academic hospital to which they primarily refer. This noticeably increases the communication between the two institutions and likely decreases medical errors and duplicated work.

Mayo Clinic in Jacksonville, Florida

One of the largest and most comprehensive team approaches at Mayo Clinic in Jacksonville, Florida, is the Cardiopulmonary Rehabilitation Program. The program utilizes many health professionals who are under the leadership of a nurse director with a physician supervisor. The team members include (but are not limited to) physical therapists, exercise specialists, dietitians, respiratory specialists, occupational therapists, and pharmacists. Patients include those who are post–myocardial infarction, post–coronary bypass surgery, post–percutaneous coronary intervention, or post-transplant. Others include high-risk subjects with coronary artery disease—that is, those with diabetes, angina, and arrhythmias—and those that are considered pre-transplant. The pulmonary component includes subjects who are post-heart/lung or lung transplantation, chronic pulmonary disease patients, and pulmonary hypertension patients. This combined program has functioned effectively for many years.

The Stress Testing Team in Cardiology at Mayo Clinic performs exercise stress testing with direct nurse supervision, and a physician is immediately available. This team of 20 to 24 nurses and other health professionals also supervises and administers the echo and stress nuclear studies and magnetic resonance stress studies. This specific team approach has been quite effective in patient care and in providing data to the responsible physician in order to choose the most appropriate mode of stress testing for a given individual.

The Heart Failure Services in cardiology at Mayo Clinic utilizes the skills of nurses and physicians to provide service to the patient. This service works closely with the heart transplant team. The service has weekly team rounds for both clinical and academic discussions.

Emphasis is made in all of the subspecialties of CVD that the role of the nurse is of vast importance to integrated team care. As the CVD residency (fellowship) has evolved at Mayo Clinic, trainees are made a part of the various aforementioned teams as their rotations permit. More interaction within the team structure fosters the teaching/learning experience. One special manifestation of this is improved patient care.

At Mayo Clinic, the importance of the scheduling and secretarial assistance to the successful team approach cannot be overlooked. The team approach could not be properly implemented if this was not in place to make the patient's and provider's roles timely, efficient, and pleasant, ensuring optimal patient outcomes.

Massachusetts General Hospital (MGH)

Outpatient Community-based Cardiac Prevention. Patients with risk factors for CVD are often hesitant to make the trip into Boston to access preventive services. For this reason, a community-based primary prevention program was developed to examine the feasibility of providing these services in a hospital-affiliated healthcare center. An example is the HAPPY Heart Study, which takes place at the MGH Revere Community Health Center. In this setting, low-income women with multiple risk factors for CVD participate in a primary prevention program. The team consists of:

- Bilingual research assistant
- Nurse health coaches
- Physical therapists

- Nutritionists
- Primary care physicians
- Supervising cardiologist

The patients who join this program are evaluated by a nurse and physical therapist and undergo routine risk factor evaluation. The cardiologist reviews the lab work and clinical data at team meetings and forwards an electronic message to the primary care physician so that adjustments of medications can be made. The patients also meet with a registered dietitian who develops an individualized plan for the patient and their family. The team works together to provide both a physical, as well as psychosocial, support network. The patients also meet as a group with the nurses twice a month for an educational presentation and interaction. This peer-to-peer interaction has proved to be an important part of the overall prevention strategy.

Cardiac Care: MGH Heart Center has developed a program-based team approach in both the inpatient and outpatient settings. Some examples of the various programs within the Heart Center include:

- Congenital Heart Disease
- Coronary Artery Disease
- Arrhythmia
- Cardiac Resynchronization
- Heart Failure and Transplantation
- Women's Heart Health
- Vascular Medicine
- Hypertrophic Cardiomyopathy
- Athlete Performance Programs

There is often close interaction between the members of the teams in the various programs, particularly in the Cardiac Resynchronization and Heart Failure Programs.

The *Heart Center Programs* each consist of teams on both the inpatient and outpatient service, with frequent overlap between members. The members of the teams include the team coordinators (administrative position), nurses, sonographers, physician assistants, and individual clinicians, including fellows and attending physicians. The patients are initially assessed by an attending physician and are then followed by other team members. Some programs include cardiologists with unique specializations.

An example of this is the *Cardiac Resynchronization Program*, which includes physicians and other healthcare professionals, representing a variety of disciplines, including the arrhythmia, heart failure, transplantation, and imaging programs. One of the key components to integrating such specialized information is the healthcare provider, who communicates with the various members and provides continuity between programs. Much of the outpatient team approach includes a virtual team approach with integration of the individual evaluations by the members of the team. As both patient acuity and the complexity of care increase, the team approach to care becomes more important. Healthcare professionals involved include nurses, nutritionists, physical therapists, psychiatrists, and pharmacists.

Another benefit of the team approach is the management of the patient with *advanced heart failure*. In this setting, the team provides the framework for the medical treatment of patients with severe heart failure and helps identify potential candidates for heart transplantation. If a patient is a candidate for heart transplantation, the same team of physicians is available both before and after transplant. The Heart Failure and Cardiac Transplant team also consult with psychiatrists and social workers who have expertise in the treatment of advanced heart disease to ease the process and relieve stressors.

The members of the team, whether attending inpatients or outpatients, are for the most part consistent; however, there are some additional members involved, depending on the diagnosis. The key members include the responding clinician (usually a house officer), the supervising physician (a cardiologist), the patient's floor nurse, an APRN or NP assigned to the specific program, a registered dietitian, a physical therapist, and a case manager. Additional members of the team who provide support as needed include an endocrinologist, nephrologist, social worker, and the palliative care APRN or NP or physician. The palliative care provider is actively involved in the management of patients with end-stage heart failure or heart failure patients who are frequently admitted and readmitted.

The continuity between the inpatient and outpatient care teams is frequently provided by the attending cardiologist. The MGH Heart Center physicians supervise their patients continuously, as there is no service model. For this reason, the complex patients are well-known by the staff at the time of the admission, a feature which can potentially minimize unnecessary testing. The cardiac patients are frequently admitted to one of three floors, and the frequently admitted patients are well-known to the nursing staff and usually cared for by familiar nurses. While the interactions of the inpatient team are usually virtual, face-to-face meetings are held when critical decisions must be made. The members of the team are familiar with one another and work well together to provide the highest level of care in the most efficient manner. The role of the case manager has become increasingly important, considering the advanced age of many of the cardiac patients and the need for safe, appropriate levels of care at the time of disposition of the patient.

Table 2
Members of Cardiac Care Teams

Services	MGH	Geisinger	Veterans Administration	Cleveland Clinic Foundation
Physician	X	X	X	X
APRN, NP, and/ or PA	X	X	X	X
Cardiac Fellow	X	X	X	X
Dietitian	X	X		
Psychologist	X	X		
Case Manager	X	X	X	X

Both Geisinger Health Systems and the Cleveland Clinic Foundation Cardiac Service line managers report that their inpatient and outpatient services were run similarly to those previously discussed. A difference between the MGH and the Cleveland Clinic models is that there is a rotating attending cardiologist caring for patients on the cardiac services at Cleveland Clinic, while at MGH, the patient's private attending or specific fellow provide continuity of care as part of the team. The inclusion of nutrition and behavioral support in the inpatient cardiac setting was emphasized in the Geisinger system (Table 2).

Roles and Responsibilities of Team Members

The CVD team can be comprised of two or more members. The integrated team works collaboratively to achieve common goals in the care of their patients. Teams are generally physician directed and nurse managed. A small clinical practice team might consist of a physician and an office co-worker, while more elaborate practice models might include (see Figure 3):

- Physician
- NP
- Clinical nurse specialist
- PA
- Dietitian
- Pharmacist
- Psychologist
- Physical therapist
- Case manager

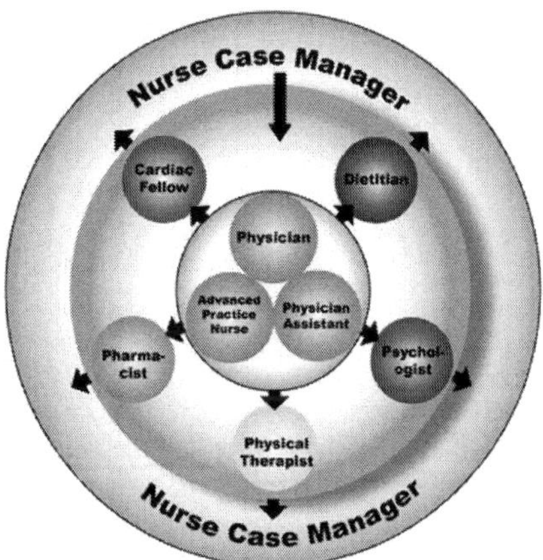

Figure 3

Integrated Team Model: An integrated team model illustrates the flow of information among the team members. This model depicts the core team of the Physician and Advanced Nurse Practitioner and/or Physician Assistant. Depending on the clinical needs of the patient, individual team members become involved based on specific needs related to their expertise. Ultimately all information reaches the Case Manager as seen by the outgoing arrows. The Case Manager ensures that everything assigned is performed. Information flows both ways, as noted by the incoming arrow from the Nurse Case Manager to the team, allowing for better patient outcomes. This is one example of an integrated team. Teams may differ from one clinical area to another.

The roles and responsibilities of each non-physician team member are based on their licensure, scope of practice, prescribing privileges, specialty certification, clinical skills and interests, and billing privileges. Considering that much of chronic care involves counseling and education, it is imperative that all team members are highly skilled in communication, understand the importance and challenges of lifestyle change, are committed to ongoing patient education, and are skilled in techniques that influence lifestyle modification, medication adherence, and self-care. Table 3 summarizes general descriptions of licensure, certification, and prescriptive privileges for selected non-physician team members. Master and doctoral degrees are offered for many healthcare professionals in their respective professions. Other non-physician healthcare team members may include:

- Psychologist
- Social worker
- Respiratory therapist
- Occupational therapist
- Physical therapist
- Spiritual/religious counselor

The Impact of Technology on Integrated Team Efforts

Technology now plays an important role in health care and makes integrated team efforts more easily implemented. For example, care of the heart failure patient is greatly facilitated by technology. Heart failure now affects nearly 5.8 million Americans and results in nearly one million hospital admissions annually. The team-based, home monitoring approach is being implemented to potentially decreased morbidity, mortality, hospital admissions, and overall cost for the treatment

Table 3

Selected Key Elements of Professional Education, Licensure, and Care Responsibilities for Certain Non-Physician Cardiovascular Team Members

Profession	Licensure	Specialty Certifications	Prescribing and Billing Privileges
Nurse Practitioner (NP)[1]	State regulated	Masters prepared. Board certification in specialty practice areas available through American Nurses Credentialing Center. Recertification is required.	Privileges differ by state. NP services include diagnosis, ordering and interpreting tests, prescribing medication, providing direct patient care, counseling and education, and health promotion and disease prevention. They can generally bill for their services. NPs work collaboratively with physicians and some work independently.
Clinical Nurse Specialist[1]	State regulated	Masters prepared. Board certification in specialty practice areas available through American Nurses Credentialing Center. Recertification is required.	Privileges differ widely by state. The Clinical Nurse Specialist is a clinical expert in a specific area of nursing practice. They provide direct patient care, diagnosis, and treatment of disease states, and are responsible for health promotion and disease prevention. Can bill for services in some states usually within a group or physician practice.
Case Manager (Generally a Registered Nurse)[2]	State regulated	May be Masters prepared. Board certification as a Case Manager is available through American Nurses Credentialing Center. Recertification is required.	Medical case managers evaluate medical status, develop and implement a plan of care, coordinate medical resources, communicate the healthcare plan with the patient and their family and coordinate care with the healthcare team. They monitor progress, plan transitions to different levels of care and plan for transition to home from hospital or sub-acute setting.
Physician Assistant[3]	State regulated	Often Masters prepared. National Commission on Certification of Physician Assistants administered by Physician Assistant National Certifying Exam; this certification is required for licensure in all states. Recertification is required.	Licensed to practice under the supervision of a physician. Privileges differ by state. Services include diagnosis, ordering and interpreting tests, prescribing medication, counseling and education, health promotion and disease prevention, and direct patient care.

continued

Table 3 *continued*

Profession	Licensure	Specialty Certifications	Prescribing and Billing Privileges
Dietitian[4]	33 states require licensure, 12 require statutory certification, and 1 requires registration.	Often Masters prepared. Commission on Dietetic Registration of the American Dietetic Association awards the Registered Dietitian credential.	Can bill for their services as part of a visit for Medical Nutrition Therapy. Coverage for their services, other than for Medical Nutrition Therapy, varies widely and is generally not covered by Medicare Part B.
Pharmacist[5]	State regulated	Often Masters prepared. The North American Pharmacist Licensure Examination is required in all states. 45 states require the Multistate Pharmacy Jurisprudence Examination.	In many team-based models of care, pharmacists play an important role in medication management, adherence, titration, and disease management programs.

Regulatory organizations

1. Consensus Model for APRN Regulation: Licensure, Accreditation, Certification & Education. Completed through the work of the APRN Consensus Work Group & the National Council of State Boards of Nursing APRN Advisory Committee. APRN Joint Dialogue Group Report, July 7, 2008. Published online and available as a pdf.
   American Nurse Credentialing Center ANCC.org
   American Academy of Nurse Practitioners AANP.org
   American College of Nurse Practitioners ACNP.org
   National Association of Clinical Nurse Specialists NACNS.org
2. Certification available through the American Nurse Credentialing Center ANCC.org
   The American Academy of Case Management AIHCP.org
   Case Management Society of America CMSA.org
3. National Commission on the Certification of Physician Assistants (NCCPA) NCCPA@NCCPA.net
   American Academy of Physician Assistants AAPA.org
4. American Dietetic Association ADA.org
   Commission on Dietetic Registration of the American Dietetic Association CDMET.org
5. North American Pharmacist Licensure Examination Multistate Pharmacy Jurisprudence Examination nabp.net/programs/examination/naplex
   American Pharmacy Alliance APA.org

of heart failure and can enhance the concept of "home-health self-care."[28] The accessibility and increased ease of use of electronic formats for patient data have revolutionized care programs. For example, MGH uses a program called Partners

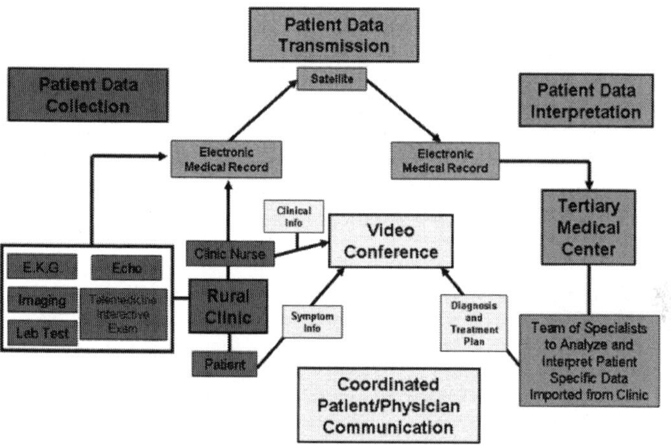

Figure 4

Telemedicine: Key elements of telemedicine care delivery programs within healthcare delivery systems are shown. These include data collection instruments, methods of data transmission, data interpretation, and integration into clinical practice through various modalities to provide optimal patient care.

Health Care Connected Cardiac Care. This program includes home-based telemonitoring and an education program for patients with heart failure who are at risk for frequent hospitalizations. Potential patients are identified and referred by hospital case managers, NPs, primary care physicians, cardiologists, and other clinicians. Following enrollment in the program, the Partners Health Care At Home telemonitoring team works with the patient by providing daily support, education, and physiologic monitoring (Figure 4).

The connected care program utilizes technology to enhance the care of the patients and to reduce the readmission rate for patients with heart failure. Vital signs and weights are measured at home, transmitted via the internet or telephone, and forwarded to their physicians. This allows for careful management of blood pressure, pulse, and weight and for the timely adjustment of medications. Patients use the provided devices to monitor their blood pressure, pulse, oxygen levels, and weight. They then utilize a touch-screen computer to answer symptom questions. This information is then transmitted to Partners Health Care At Home. A nurse reviews the data, and appropriate intervention is taken when readings are outside of established ranges. This includes a call to the patient to determine what caused the change and what is necessary to return to normal. Advantages of this approach include the ability to provide this service in the patient's own environment. Daily monitoring coupled with structured weekly education sessions helps patients to become keenly aware of their daily behaviors and of the impact this has on their condition. Patients learn that specific interventions do make a difference. This results in behavior changes and the development of new self-management skills. When patients are not within proper range, collaboration with clinicians in real time often results in prompt intervention and avoidance of emergency department visits or hospitalization. A favorable aspect is that the patients surveyed reported that this process improved their understanding of heart failure and their confidence—both of which help minimize hospitalizations.

Flagstaff, Arizona, Hospital recently launched a program entitled "Care Beyond Walls and Wires," which is partially sponsored by the National Institutes of Health, Verizon Wireless, and Zephyr Technology. Upon discharge, the patients are provided with a home monitoring package that includes a Motorola Droid X2 smart phone, an app for transmitting patient data, monitors for oxygen saturation, heart rate, and tracking programs for blood pressure as well as weight. Data is transmitted to a team of clinicians who follow data and track adherence and clinical status. The type of monitoring should alert both physicians and patients of a potential impending heart failure exacerbation. Additional technological enhancements include computer programs and applications for smart phones.

Hundreds of applications now available can be used to manage CVD. These applications allow the patient and their healthcare provider to work together to better manage their care. Applications are available to measure blood pressure and heart rate.

Cost-effectiveness and the Team-based Approach

In 2008, the Healthcare Cost and Utilization Project reported on potentially preventable hospitalizations for acute and chronic conditions. These preventable chronic conditions were defined as diabetes, specific respiratory conditions, and specific circulatory conditions. Sixty percent of hospitalizations were for persons 65 years of age and older, in persons of lower socio-economic status, and in the uninsured.[29] This report found that 1 out of every 10 hospital stays was preventable for acute and chronic conditions. This clearly demonstrates the importance of implementing risk reduction strategies to reduce the incidence of preventable conditions. Physical activity, following a heart healthy diet, maintaining a normal body weight, cessation of smoking, and management of high blood cholesterol, Type 2 diabetes, and hypertension are all key risk reduction strategies. In concert, they play a significantly important role in reducing preventable hospitalizations.[30-32]

Cardiovascular disease, generally a result of well-defined and preventable risk factors, is the leading cause of death in adult Americans, irrespective of gender, with the largest percentage of deaths occurring in persons over 65 years of age. The American Heart Association lists cigarette smoking, high blood pressure, high blood cholesterol, and physical inactivity as the top four modifiable risks for coronary heart disease.[18,19] Additionally, the risk of developing of Type 2 diabetes in adults with elevated fasting blood glucose can be reduced by 58% with intensive nutrition, weight loss, and physical activity in adults.[20] One report examined the effects of achieving nationally recommended prevention goals on CVD-related morbidity, mortality, Quality Adjusted Life Years saved, and cost of these activities in the United States. They predicted, based on their evaluation model, that "if every person could receive the prevention goals for which he or she is a candidate, myocardial infarction could be reduced ~60% (from ~43 million over 30 years to ~16 million), strokes could be reduced 30% (from ~33 million over 30 years to ~23 million), and everyone's life expectancies could be increased an average of 1.3 years and at a higher quality of life than currently experienced."[24]

"Improving Primary Care for Patients with Chronic Illness" examined 27 studies. They found that 18 of 27 prior studies examining a more team-based chronic healthcare management program in patients with chronic conditions led to reduced utilization of healthcare services and lower healthcare costs in patients with common chronic health conditions including heart failure, asthma, and diabetes.[33]

Another group examined the effectiveness of a comprehensive, multidisciplinary team approach on reduction in hospital readmissions in patients with heart failure. They randomized 200 patients hospitalized to participate in a multidisciplinary program or usual care. The multidisciplinary team consisted of a cardiologist, a heart failure nurse, a telephone nurse coordinator, and the patient's primary physician. The patient's medications were adjusted according to an algorithm calculated by the nurse. While costs were similar in both groups, the intervention group enjoyed improved quality of life, higher likelihood of achieving target vasodilator dose, and improved dietary compliance. There were fewer admissions in the intervention group, although this did not meet statistical significance.[34]

Another report consisted of a meta-analysis of 19 randomized controlled clinical trials (5,752 patients). This meta-analysis evaluated the heart failure disease management programs, examined all-cause hospitalization, and demonstrated a decrease in all-cause hospitalization for the patients in the intervention groups.[35]

The ability to clearly demonstrate the cost-effectiveness of team-based care of the cardiac patient is a complex task due to the multiple variables involved in such an analysis. The members of the team, inpatient or outpatient status, and acuity of the patient all influence cost and potential outcomes. Interdisciplinary care has been demonstrated to favorably affect quality and duration of life, as well as a reduction in readmissions to the hospital. Further work needs to be done to more clearly define the cost benefits of team care.

Patient Education, Health Literacy, and the Team Approach

Patient education is vital to improving clinical outcomes in CVD patients. This is usually done by the team physician stressing the need for behavior change or medication adherence and the nurse and other appropriate team members providing in-depth patient education.

Health literacy is the ability to obtain, process, and understand health information and make appropriate health decisions.[36] In the United States, adults can be divided into four levels of general literacy and math tasks:

- Below basic
- Basic
- Intermediate
- Proficient

Of these four levels, 43% of adults function at below basic and basic, and 44% function at the intermediate level of general literacy skills.[37] This is important, since many adults functioning at the intermediate and proficient levels of general literacy function at lower levels of health literacy.[37] In fact, 88% of American adults have health literacy skills below proficient.[38] Low health literacy adds an annual cost to the healthcare system of $106 to $238 billion.[39] Thus, the Joint Commission now requires patient education materials to be at or below a 5th grade reading level and "in clear or plain language" that the patient can understand.[40,41]

Patients with low health literacy are three times more likely to experience adverse health problems.[42] Patients with lower health literacy and a chronic condition, such as cardiovascular disease, are at increased risk for poor health outcomes, including poor self-care, frequent medication errors, increased hospitalizations, and increased mortality.[43-47]

Many physicians and nurses assume their patients are functionally literate and communicate with patients while assuming they can read and comprehend information. The healthcare team is often rushed, making the patient feel rushed or uncomfortable, and the patient may be too embarrassed to ask questions that may result in the exposure of his or her limited literacy skills.[48] The goal with patient education is to help the patient become informed and engaged. The team should create an open environment in which the patient feels comfortable to ask questions.[48]

Patients with limited health literacy have poor diabetic control;[49] often present with more advanced diseases, such as prostate cancer;[50] use fewer preventive services;[51] and are twice as likely to be hospitalized.[46] Additionally, older adults with limited health literacy have a hazard ratio for mortality over a 5-year period of 1.52 compared with those with normal health literacy.[47] Many factors account for this poor health status, including:

- Increasingly complex healthcare system
- Difficulties accessing health care

- Limitations in patient-provider communication
- Failure of providers to promote self-management
- Failure to recognize patient barriers to communication and comprehension[52]

As the health team encourages the patient and family to become more proactive and to utilize self-care in the management of their cardiovascular disease, communication becomes paramount, whether delivered verbally or in written patient education materials. For better patient outcomes, keep it simple. Key points for written and verbal communication and patient education materials are highlighted in Table 4 and Table 5.

Table 4
Key Points for Patient Education Written Materials[53]

Sentence Structure	• Large letters: 13–16 type font • Short words and short sentences • Give examples to explain difficult words
The Message	• Include interaction • Repeat important information • Avoid medical jargon; i.e., CT scan • Key behavioral information should be first to build self-efficacy • Explain purpose or benefit at the beginning
Page Layout	• Keep ample "white space" on each page to avoid look of all text • Use headers to introduce new topics or break up page • Use lowercase rather than UPPERCASE • Keep left margin even and right uneven • Lists should be no more than 5 • Realistic photos better than cartoons • Best colors are yellow, green, and white

Table 5
Key Points for Written or Verbal Communication[48]

Context First vs. Last	
"You can lose weight if you eat less animal fat and sugar." "Reducing animal fat and sugars as well as including more fiber can help in weight loss."	
Communicate in the Active Voice	
"Weigh yourself every morning as soon as you get out of bed." (Active)	"Weights should be recorded first thing each morning." (Passive)
Simple vs. Formal Communication Style	
"When your cholesterol is above 200, you need a pill." (Simple)	"Sometimes your blood cholesterol may be too high and your diet is not effective. In cases like this...." (Formal)

Concluding Remarks

It is imperative that healthcare providers continue to research and implement efficient and cost-effective integrated team-based care. This type of care has been shown to improve quality of life and reduce morbidity and mortality. Creating systematic approaches to care holds the promise of making these services cost-effective for individual patients and society as a whole.

In this discussion, emphasis has been on the role of the integrated healthcare team in the management of the patient with CVD. It should be noted that the patient likely has his or her "personal team" of family and friends with whom the healthcare team must effectively relate during the transition from hospital to home. Examples could be the person who provides food and beverage for the patient, the one who ensures proper administration of medications, the one responsible for coordinating delivery of medical supplies, or the one who coordinates device checking or monitoring. All of these supplementary "patient team" members must work closely with the healthcare team member who has skills in these specific subsets.

With this collaborative approach to patient care and with adherence to established practice guidelines, optimal patient outcomes can be achieved with cost-effectiveness. The details in the previous discussions provide the reader with practical information to effectively implement the integrated team approach in the care of the patient with CVD.

Acknowledgments: The authors would like to thank Victoria L. Jackson, MLIS (Academic and Research Support, Mayo Clinic, Jacksonville, Florida) for her editorial support and assistance on this project.

REFERENCES

1. Berra K. Childrearing women and their families: setting the stage for heart health. *Cardiol Rev*. Mar-Apr 2011;19(2):66–70. http://www.ncbi.nlm.nih.gov/pubmed/21285665.
2. Schwandt P, Haas GM, Liepold E. Lifestyle and cardiovascular risk factors in 2001 child-parent pairs: the PEP Family Heart Study. *Atherosclerosis*. Dec 2010;213(2):642–648. http://www.ncbi.nlm.nih.gov/pubmed/20980001.
3. Kavey RE, Daniels SR, Lauer RM, Atkins DL, Hayman LL, Taubert K. American Heart Association guidelines for primary prevention of atherosclerotic cardiovascular disease beginning in childhood. *Circulation*. Mar 25 2003;107(11):1562–1566. http://www.ncbi.nlm.nih.gov/pubmed/12654618.
4. Lyons AS, Petrucelli RJ. *Medicine: An Illustrated History*. New York: H. N. Abrams Inc.; 1978.
5. Fletcher GF, Cantwell JD. Outpatient gym exercise program for patients with recent myocardial infarction. A preliminary report. *Arch Intern Med*. Jul 1974;134(1):63–68. http://www.ncbi.nlm.nih.gov/pubmed/4833934.
6. Fletcher GF, Cantwell JD. Ventricular fibrillation in a medically supervised cardiac exercise program. Clinical, angiographic, and surgical correlations. *JAMA*. 1977;238(24):2627–2629.

7. Fletcher GF, Cantwell JD, Watt EW. Oxygen consumption and hemodynamic response of exercises used in training of patients with recent myocardial infarction. *Circulation*. Jul 1979;60(1):140–144. http://www.ncbi.nlm.nih.gov/pubmed/445716.
8. Oldridge NB, Guyatt GH, Fischer ME, Rimm AA. Cardiac rehabilitation after myocardial infarction. Combined experience of randomized clinical trials. *JAMA*. 1988;260(7):945–950.
9. Hartley LH. Exercise and cardiac rehabilitation. *Proc N Engl Cardiovasc Soc*. 1976;28:37–40.
10. Redwood DR, Rosing DR, Epstein SE. Circulatory and symptomatic effects of physical training in patients with coronary artery disease and angina pectoris. *N Engl J Med*. 1972;286(18):959–965.
11. DeBusk RF, Haskell WL, Miller NH, et al. Medically directed at-home rehabilitation soon after clinically uncomplicated acute myocardial infarction: a new model for patient care. *Am J Cardiol*. 1985;55(4):251–257.
12. Institute of Medicine, Committee on Quality of Health Care in America. *Crossing the Quality Chasm: A New Health System for the 21st Century*. Washington, DC: National Academy Press; 2001.
13. Wagner EH, Austin BT, Von Korff M. Improving outcomes in chronic illness. *Manag Care Q*. Spring 1996;4(2):12–25. http://www.ncbi.nlm.nih.gov/pubmed/10157259.
14. Wagner EH, Davis C, Schaefer J, Von Korff M, Austin B. A survey of leading chronic disease management programs: are they consistent with the literature? *Manag Care Q*. Summer 1999;7(3):56–66. http://www.ncbi.nlm.nih.gov/pubmed/10620960.
15. DeBusk RF, Miller NH, Superko HR, et al. A case-management system for coronary risk factor modification after acute myocardial infarction. *Ann Intern Med*. 1994;120(9):721–729.
16. Haskell WL, Alderman EL, Fair JM, et al. Effects of intensive multiple risk factor reduction on coronary atherosclerosis and clinical cardiac events in men and women with coronary artery disease. The Stanford Coronary Risk Intervention Project (SCRIP). *Circulation*. 1994;89(3):975–990.
17. Wood DA, Kotseva K, Connolly S, et al. Nurse-coordinated multidisciplinary, family-based cardiovascular disease prevention programme (EUROACTION) for patients with coronary heart disease and asymptomatic individuals at high risk of cardiovascular disease: a paired, cluster-randomised controlled trial. *Lancet*. Jun 14 2008;371(9629):1999–2012. http://www.ncbi.nlm.nih.gov/pubmed/18555911.
18. Berra K. Does nurse case management improve implementation of guidelines for cardiovascular disease risk reduction? *J Cardiovasc Nurs*. 2011;26(2):145–167.

19. Fonarow GC, Gawlinski A, Moughrabi S, Tillisch JH. Improved treatment of coronary heart disease by implementation of a Cardiac Hospitalization Atherosclerosis Management Program (CHAMP). *Am J Cardiol.* Apr 1 2001;87(7):819–822. http://www.ncbi.nlm.nih.gov/pubmed/11274933.

20. Bayliss EA, Edwards AE, Steiner JF, Main DS. Processes of care desired by elderly patients with multimorbidities. *Fam Pract.* Aug 2008;25(4):287–293. http://www.ncbi.nlm.nih.gov/pubmed/18628243.

21. Boult C, Green AF, Boult LB, Pacala JT, Snyder C, Leff B. Successful models of comprehensive care for older adults with chronic conditions: evidence for the Institute of Medicine's "retooling for an aging America" report. *J Am Geriatr Soc.* Dec 2009;57(12):2328–2337. http://www.ncbi.nlm.nih.gov/pubmed/20121991.

22. Lin EH, Von Korff M, Ciechanowski P, et al. Treatment adjustment and medication adherence for complex patients with diabetes, heart disease, and depression: a randomized controlled trial. *Ann Fam Med.* Jan 2012;10(1):6–14. http://www.ncbi.nlm.nih.gov/pubmed/22230825.

23. Boult C, Reider L, Leff B, et al. The effect of guided care teams on the use of health services: results from a cluster-randomized controlled trial. *Arch Intern Med.* Mar 14 2011;171(5):460–466. http://www.ncbi.nlm.nih.gov/pubmed/21403043.

24. Kahn R, Robertson RM, Smith R, Eddy D. The impact of prevention on reducing the burden of cardiovascular disease. *Circulation.* Jul 29 2008;118(5):576–585. http://www.ncbi.nlm.nih.gov/pubmed/18606915.

25. About VHA. *United States: Department of Veterans Affairs.* 2011. http://www.va.gov/health/aboutVHA.asp.

26. National Center for Veterans Analysis and Statistics. *United States Department of Veterans Affairs.* 2010. http://www.va.gov/vetdata/.

27. Jha AK, DesRoches CM, Campbell EG, et al. Use of electronic health records in U.S. hospitals. *N Engl J Med.* Apr 16 2009;360(16):1628–1638. http://www.ncbi.nlm.nih.gov/pubmed/19321858.

28. Bui AL, Fonarow GC. Home monitoring for heart failure management. *J Am Coll Cardiol.* Jan 10 2012;59(2):97–104. http://www.ncbi.nlm.nih.gov/pubmed/22222071.

29. Stranges E, Stocks C. *Potentially Preventable Hospitalizations for Acute and Chronic Conditions, 2008*: Statistical Brief #99. Feb 2006. http://www.ncbi.nlm.nih.gov/pubmed/21413210.

30. Roger VL, Go AS, Lloyd-Jones DM, et al. Heart disease and stroke statistics—2011 update: a report from the American Heart Association. *Circulation.* Feb 1 2011;123(4):e18–e209. http://www.ncbi.nlm.nih.gov/pubmed/21160056.

31. Understand Your Risk of Heart Attack. 2011; http://www.heart.org/HEARTORG/Conditions/HeartAttack/UnderstandYourRiskof-HeartAttack/Understand-Your-Risk-of-Heart-Attack_UCM_002040_Article.jsp.
32. Knowler WC, Barrett-Connor E, Fowler SE, et al. Reduction in the incidence of type 2 diabetes with lifestyle intervention or metformin. *N Engl J Med.* Feb 7 2002;346(6):393–403. http://www.ncbi.nlm.nih.gov/entrez/query.fcgi?cmd=Retrieve&db=PubMed&dopt=Citation&list_uids=11832527.
33. Bodenheimer T, Wagner EH, Grumbach K. Improving primary care for patients with chronic illness: the chronic care model, Part 2. *JAMA.* Oct 16 2002;288(15):1909–1914. http://www.ncbi.nlm.nih.gov/pubmed/12377092.
34. Kasper EK, Gerstenblith G, Hefter G, et al. A randomized trial of the efficacy of multidisciplinary care in heart failure outpatients at high risk of hospital readmission. *J Am Coll Cardiol.* Feb 6 2002;39(3):471–480. http://www.ncbi.nlm.nih.gov/pubmed/11823086.
35. Whellan DJ, Hasselblad V, Peterson E, O'Connor CM, Schulman KA. Meta-analysis and review of heart failure disease management randomized controlled clinical trials. *Am Heart J.* Apr 2005;149(4):722–729. http://www.ncbi.nlm.nih.gov/pubmed/15990759.
36. *Healthy People 2000.* Centers for Disease Control and Prevention. 2000. http://www.cdc.gov/nchs/healthy_people/hp2000.htm.
37. *National Assessment of Adult Literacy (NAAL).* National Center for Education Statistics. 2003. http://nces.ed.gov/naal/.
38. *The Health Literacy of America's Adults: Results from the 2003 National Assessment of Adult Literacy.* National Center for Education Statistics. 2006. http://nces.ed.gov/pubsearch/pubsinfo.asp?pubid=2006483.
39. Debuono B. *Low Health Literacy: Implications for National Policy.* 2007. http://www.gwumc.edu/sphhs/departments/healthpolicy/chsrp/downloads/LowHealthLiteracyReport10_4_07.pdf.
40. The Joint Commission. *"What did the doctor say?" Improving health literacy to protect patient safety.* Health Care at the Crossroads Reports. 2007.
41. The Joint Commission. *Advancing effective communication, cultural competence, and patient- and family-centered care: A roadmap for hospitals.* The Joint Commission. 2010.
42. Dewalt DA, Berkman ND, Sheridan S, Lohr KN, Pignone MP. Literacy and health outcomes: a systematic review of the literature. *J Gen Intern Med.* Dec 2004;19(12):1228–1239. http://www.ncbi.nlm.nih.gov/pubmed/15610334.

43. Baker DW, Gazmararian JA, Williams MV, et al. Functional health literacy and the risk of hospital admission among Medicare managed care enrollees. *Am J Public Health.* Aug 2002;92(8):1278–1283. http://www.ncbi.nlm.nih.gov/pubmed/12144984.
44. Gazmararian JA, Williams MV, Peel J, Baker DW. Health literacy and knowledge of chronic disease. *Patient Educ Couns.* Nov 2003;51(3):267–275. http://www.ncbi.nlm.nih.gov/pubmed/14630383.
45. Berkman ND, Sheridan SL, Donahue KE, et al. *Health Literacy Interventions and Outcomes: An Updated Systematic Review.* Agency for Healthcare Research and Quality. 2011. http://www.ahrq.gov/downloads/pub/evidence/pdf/literacy/literacyup.pdf.
46. Baker DW, Parker RM, Williams MV, Clark WS. Health literacy and the risk of hospital admission. *J Gen Intern Med.* Dec 1998;13(12):791–798. http://www.ncbi.nlm.nih.gov/pubmed/9844076.
47. Baker DW, Wolf MS, Feinglass J, Thompson JA, Gazmararian JA, Huang J. Health literacy and mortality among elderly persons. *Arch Intern Med.* Jul 23 2007;167(14):1503–1509. http://www.ncbi.nlm.nih.gov/pubmed/17646604.
48. Oates DJ, Paasche-Orlow MK. Health literacy: communication strategies to improve patient comprehension of cardiovascular health. *Circulation.* Feb 24 2009;119(7):1049–1051. http://www.ncbi.nlm.nih.gov/pubmed/19237675.
49. Schillinger D, Grumbach K, Piette J, et al. Association of health literacy with diabetes outcomes. *JAMA.* Jul 24–31 2002;288(4):475–482. http://www.ncbi.nlm.nih.gov/pubmed/12132978.
50. Bennett CL, Ferreira NR, Davis TC, et al. Relationship between literacy, race and stage of presentation among low income patients with prostate cancer. *J Clin Oncol.* 1998;16:3101–3104.
51. Scott TL, Gazmararian JA, Williams MV, Baker DW. Health literacy and preventive health care use among Medicare enrollees in a managed care organization. *Med Care.* May 2002;40(5):395–404. http://www.ncbi.nlm.nih.gov/pubmed/11961474.
52. Paasche-Orlow MK, Parker RM. Improving the effectiveness of patient education: a focus on limited health literacy. In: King TE, Wheeler M, Fernandez A, eds. *Medical Management of Vulnerable and Underserved Patients: Principles, Practice and Populations.* New York: McGraw-Hill; 2007.
53. Doak CC, Doak LG, Root JH. *Teaching Patients with Low Literacy Skills.* 2 ed. Philadelphia: JB Lippincott Company; 1996.

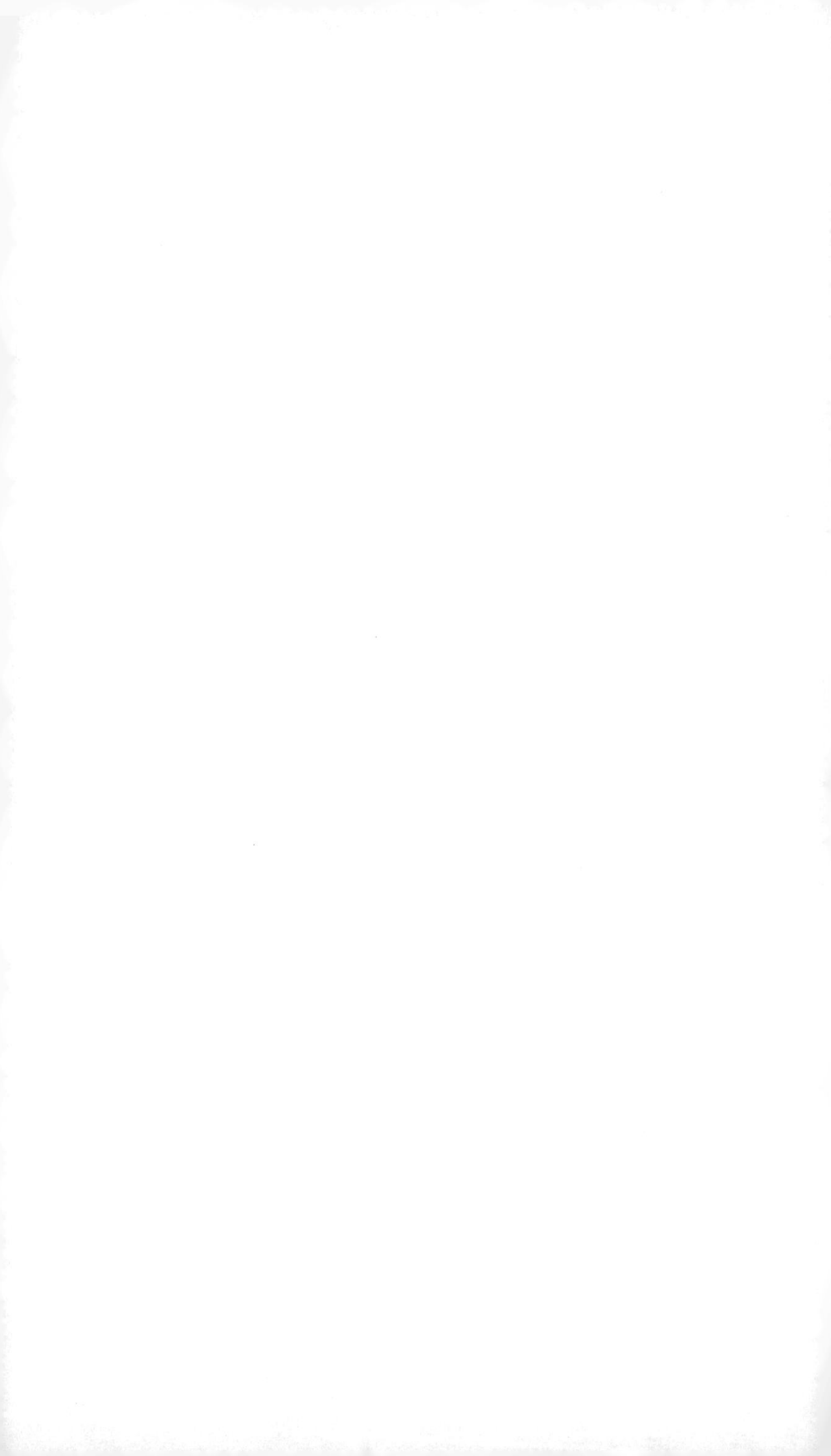

Section I

The Syndrome of Heart Failure

CHAPTER 1

The Basics

Ileana L. Piña, MD, MPH and
Elizabeth A. Madigan, PhD, RN

EPIDEMIOLOGY

Heart failure (HF) occurs when the heart is unable to meet the metabolic requirements of organ systems at normal blood pressures. HF is a syndrome and the end stage of multiple etiologies, such as hypertension, coronary artery disease (CAD), cardiomyopathy, and valvular heart disease. The incidence of HF increases among populations of increasing age and, as the United States becomes "grayer," the number of HF patients will continue to grow.[1] However, even younger subjects can suffer from HF. Symptoms that prevail during HF are dyspnea on exertion, fatigue, and volume (fluid) retention. The life expectancy and quality of life are adversely affected in these groups, and hospitalizations result from the burden of HF-related morbidity.

In the United States, the prevalence of HF has continued to increase for both Medicare recipients and HMO and insurance participants.[2] Unfortunately, and, compounding this epidemic, although great advances have been made in medical therapy for HF and other cardiovascular syndromes, a chasm exists between what is best evidence-based care and what occurs in actual practice. New cases of HF have increased to more than a total of 600,000 per year. In fact, HF constitutes the number-one discharge diagnosis in the United States for Medicare beneficiaries, accounting for more than 700,000 admissions yearly at a cost of $24.3 billion: 5.4% of total U.S. healthcare costs.[3-5] Figure 1.1 shows the increase in HF hospitalizations.

Heart Failure: Strategies to Improve Outcomes © 2013 Joseph S. Alpert, Lynne T. Braun, Barbara J. Fletcher, Gerald Fletcher, Editors-in-chief. Cardiotext Publishing, ISBN: 978-1-935395-50-8.

Figure 1.1

Trends in Heart Failure Hospitalizations

Source: Fang et al; *J Am Coll Cardiol.* 2008;52:428–434.

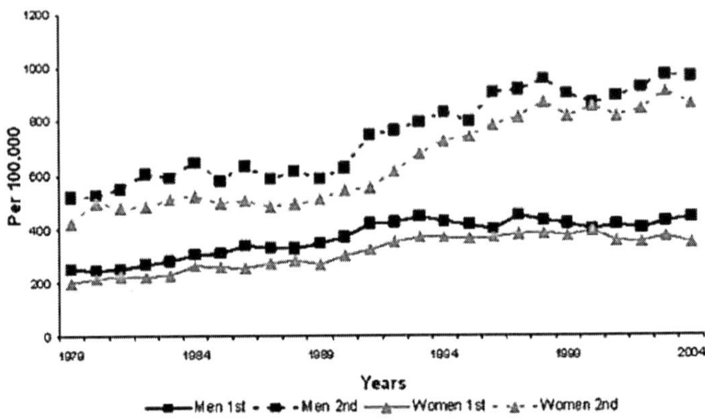

HF is not only the number one reason for hospitalization of Medicare recipients but also the major cause of 30-day re-hospitalizations.[6] Approximately 20% of patients who are discharged after an exacerbation of HF return to the hospital within 30 days. Some evidence shows that this number has increased and is associated with an ever-shrinking length of stay. Although inpatient mortality is low, once hospitalized, the outlook for those patients worsens so that mortality can be as high as 30% in one year.[7] This high mortality rate is in sharp contrast to that of symptomatic HF patients in clinical trials, which can be as low as 8%.[8]

CAUSES, NATURAL HISTORY, AND PROGNOSIS

HF can be described in various ways, as shown in Table 1.1. Systolic HF implies low ejection fraction (EF) due to loss of myocardium, as in a myocardial infarction (MI) or owing to pathology of the muscle itself (eg, cardiomyopathy). Systolic dysfunction is a defect in the ability of heart myofibrils to shorten in response to increased load. Systolic dysfunction can exist in asymptomatic individuals as well.

Table 1.1
Forms of Heart Failure

Forms of Heart Failure
• Systolic HFREF (heart failure with reduced ejection fraction)
• Diastolic HFpEF (heart failure with preserved ejection fraction)
• High-output failure Pregnancy, anemia, thyrotoxicosis, arteriovenous (AV) fistula, beriberi, Paget's disease
• Low-output failure—most common
• Acute Examples: large MI, aortic valve dysfunction
• Chronic—most common
• Right- vs. left-sided heart failure: Causes of right-sided heart failure: Left-sided failure Pulmonary embolism Pulmonary hypertension Right ventricular (RV) infarction

HF due to diastolic dysfunction, also known as heart failure with preserved ejection fraction (HFpEF), is defined as impaired left ventricular (LV) filling at normal left atrial pressure. It is more common in the elderly, particularly women, and today accounts for approximately 40% of admissions for HF. (Note that many patients have both systolic and diastolic dysfunction.) Currently, we do not have the ideal therapy for HFpEF, and clinical trials of various drugs have not shown that they result in any consistent improvement in morbidity or mortality.[9-10] Recommendations for treatment will be discussed below.

Other descriptors of HF include high output failure, which has specific causes, including AV fistulas and anemia, among others. In the healthcare setting, acute HF as an initial presentation is not as common as an acute exacerbation of a chronic state of HF. The causes of HF are shown in Table 1.2. These include ischemic disease, hypertension, and valvular disorders, among others.

Table 1.2 Common Etiologies of Heart Failure
• Ischemic heart disease
• Hypertensive heart disease
• Idiopathic cardiomyopathy
• Valvular heart disease
• Specific cardiomyopathy (eg, alcoholic, postpartum, hereditary, adriamycin)
• Myocarditis

The mortality of HF patients is associated with their clinical status, as described by New York Heart Association (NYHA) classes I–IV, but can also be affected by comorbidities such as diabetes or renal disease. Untreated class IV patients have a mortality of 50% in 6 months.[11] In clinical trials of class II–III patients, annual mortality rates can be as low as 8%.[12] However, once patients are hospitalized, their mortality rate increases to as high as 30% in 1 year.[13]

PATHOPHYSIOLOGY

HF is the last stage of the cardiovascular continuum shown in Figure 1.2. Stage A refers to patients with risk factors for HF but no evidence of ventricular dysfunction. Stage B indicates a point at which changes in ventricular function have already

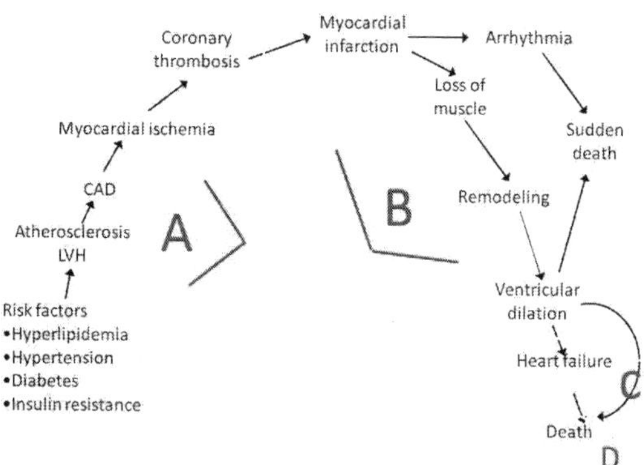

Figure 1.2

From Risk Factors to Heart Failure: The Cardiovascular Continuum

Source: Adapted from Dzau and Braunwald. *Am Heart J.* 1991;131:1244–1263.

occurred but the patient remains asymptomatic. Therefore, stage B indicates that cardiac remodeling has already occurred. Regardless of the insult (eg, MI), in HF the ventricle both hypertrophies and dilates, and the sympathetic nervous system is stimulated by increased production of norepinephrine and, ultimately, epinephrine. These systems are initially compensatory reactions to restore heart functioning but ultimately fail or overcompensate, resulting in volume expansion and further worsening ventricular dysfunction. Remodeling may take years to occur, during which changes in ventricular function are occurring but the patient remains largely asymptomatic. Stages C and D are reached when symptoms appear, such as dyspnea on exertion and fluid volume retention.[16]

The neurohormonal cascade concentrates on the deleterious effects of angiotensin II (AII), a peptide resulting from the effects of angiotensin-converting enzyme (ACE) on angiotensin I, which is produced by the actions of renin on the

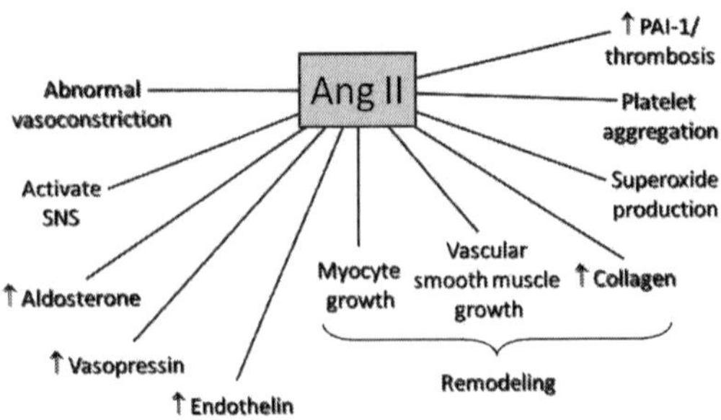

Figure 1.3

Deleterious Effects of Angiotensin II

PAI-1 = plasminogen activator inhibitor-1; SNS = sympathetic nervous system.

Source: Adapted from Burnier M, Brunner HR. *Lancet*. 2000;355: 637–645. Brown NJ, Vaughan DE. *Adv Inter Med*. 2000;45:419–429.

pro-peptide angiotensinogen. Figure 1.3 illustrates the multiple pathways that AII's actions follow, including stimulating vasopressin, aldosterone, and endothelin, as well as affecting remodeling and the clotting cascade. Most cardiovascular disease (CVD) drugs used today act on this pathway, which is known as the renin-angiotensin-aldosterone system (RAAS).

TAKING PATIENT HISTORY

The importance of taking a complete patient history in HF cannot be overemphasized. The most common presentation of HF is dyspnea, which initially occurs on exertion but gradually progresses to become a symptom at rest. Ultimately, the patient will complain of orthopnea and perhaps cough at night when recumbent. The other most frequent complaint is that of fatigue that noticeably limits activities. In addition, early satiety, abdominal fullness, and peripheral edema can present as symptoms. A history should be detailed and take into account the time since symptom development and progression. Factors that contribute to decompensation should also be reviewed. These include, but are not limited to, nonadherence to medications or diet; addition of medications that worsen LV function (eg, nonsteroidal agents or NSAIDs); removal or suboptimal use of guideline-based therapies (eg, ACE inhibitors); upper respiratory infections (URIs); anemia; and arrhythmias.[17] Other subtle signs may include persistent symptoms of URI, asthma, bronchitis, nausea and vomiting, and inability to concentrate. Often decompensation episodes follow similar patterns, such as nonadherence to limitations on sodium intake. In fact, even when medication regimens are optimized, nonadherence to a low sodium diet can lead to decompensation.[18]

Physical Examination

The physical examination should primarily include an assessment of volume and output. Presentations can be divided into several categories: "wet and warm" (the most common),[19] referring to volume overload but preserved output; "wet and cold," referring to volume overload and impaired output, resulting in peripheral vasoconstriction; and "dry and cold," which implies volume depletion with vasoconstriction. Table 1.3 depicts aspects of output and volume assessment. Low cardiac output can result in an abnormally narrowed pulse pressure, peripheral vasoconstriction with cool extremities, and low urine output.

Table 1.3 The Physical Examination
• Cardiac output Extremities Pulse pressure Mental acuity Fatigue Low urine output
• Volume Jugular venous pressure; hepatojugular reflux Chest Cardiac gallops, murmurs Hepatomegaly, ascites Edema

Volume excess can present with high jugular venous pressure (JVP), edema, pulmonary crackles, abdominal distension due to ascites or hepatic congestion, and cardiac gallops or murmurs. Adequately assessing JVP, although not a perfect indicator, can assist in evaluating changes in volume in a patient that is followed longitudinally. Figure 1.4 illustrates the measurement of JVP.

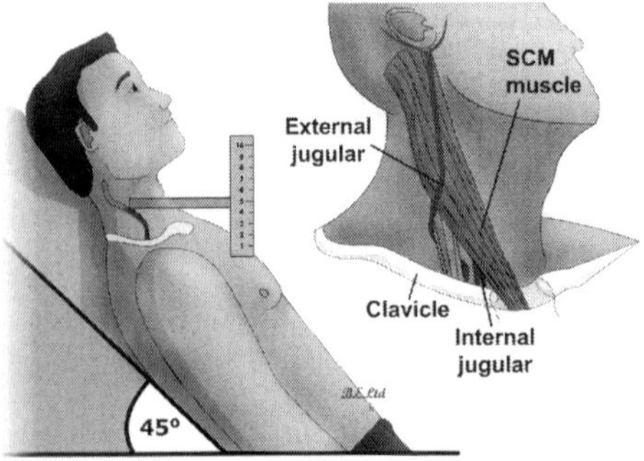

Figure 1.4

Measurement of jugular venous pressure

Source: With permission from Bloomsbury Educational Ltd.

LABORATORY TESTING

Laboratory testing should include baseline assessments of electrolytes, BUN, creatinine, complete blood count (CBC), and liver function enzymes. Furthermore, glomerular filtration rate (GFR) should be estimated as a more accurate determination of renal function than creatinine. A thyroid function panel will help in ruling out hypothyroidism as a cause of HF that can be treated with supplemental thyroid hormone. Although the total story surrounding brain natriuretic peptide (BNP) has not been elucidated, it is reasonable to obtain at least one BNP measurement during the course of therapy to rule out other causes of dyspnea.[20] Should the values for BNP be less than 100 pg/mL, it is possible that the symptoms are not related to the heart. It is widely recognized, however, that a discharge BNP that has not decreased during an admission for decompensation is a marker of future events, including rehospitalization.[21] A study by Januzzi and colleagues followed serially increasing NT-proBNP readings with augmented therapies, including aldosterone inhibitors, ACE inhibitors, and other agents, resulting in an impressive reduction in events. However, this study was small and needs replication in a larger and more diverse population.[22] The reader is referred to other, more extensive readings on this subject.[23-24]

THERAPEUTIC OPTIONS

Medical therapy for HF includes ACE inhibitors (ACEIs), angiotensin II receptor blockers (ARBs), beta (β) blockers, diuretics, and spironolactone. Device therapy includes biventricular pacing and implantable cardioverter–defibrillators (ICDs) for preventing arrhythmias and sudden death. Education and frequent monitoring are also strongly recommended, along with sodium restriction, activity recommendations, ideal weight achievement, and, for smokers, smoking cessation. As a patient's condition worsens, mechanical circulatory assistance and transplantation become options for a small percentage. Other patients and families benefit from palliative and hospice care at end of life.[25-26]

Medical Therapy

Given that there are no proven mortality-reducing therapies for HFpEF, the recommendations discussed here are relevant to HF with reduced ejection fraction (HFREF). The American College of Cardiology/American Heart Association (ACC/AHA) Guidelines clearly state that ACEIs are the first line of therapy in patients with HFREF for reducing both mortality and morbidity. ACEIs decrease AII levels by blocking the converting enzyme that results in the formation of AII from angiotensin I. In this fashion, ACEIs also block the downstream effects of AII, which include the production of aldosterone and vasopressin. Early studies of ACEIs in the treatment of HF included both patients with NYHA class IV symptoms and less ill patients with NYHA class II–III symptoms.[27-29] These studies showed a reduction in mortality and, in the case of the class II–III patients, a drop in hospitalization rates and disease progression.[30-31] The use of ACEIs serves as a way of measuring performance for both Medicare and The Joint Commission because it is linked to favorable outcomes. If the patient is truly ACEI intolerant (eg, develops angioedema or intractable cough), an ARB is a reasonable alternative. ARBs differ from ACEIs by blocking the AII and AT1 receptor directly, with downstream effects similar to those of the ACEIs.[14,15] The ARBs valsartan and candesartan were studied in a population of patients not taking ACEIs, with positive results.[32-33] At this time, only valsartan and candesartan are approved by the FDA for the HF indication. For both of these agents, it is important to titrate the doses upward to the levels recommended in the ACC/AHA Guidelines.[34]

The next line of therapy is the use of β blockers. Previously, β blockers had been feared in the treatment of HF owing to their inherent negative inotropic characteristics. However, reports in the 1990s consistently showed the deleterious effects of the secretion of catecholamines, which not only characterizes HF but worsens ventricular function.[35-36] Carefully performed trials began to amass a large body of data showing the benefits of administering β blockers in HF, not only for reducing mortality but also for reversing remodeling due to ventricular dilatation.[37-39] Three agents have shown proven improvements in mortality, morbidity, and, in some cases, reduction of sudden death in addition to reversing ventricle remodeling. These are carvedilol, metoprolol succinate (long acting), and bisoprolol.[40-42] Similar to the regimens for ACEIs and ARBs, β blockers need to be gradually up-titrated to the doses recommended in the ACC/AHA Guidelines. See Tables 1.4A and 1.4B.[43,44]

Data are emerging in the HF literature concerning the negative effects of diuretics in patients with HF. Among the arguments for limiting diuretic use in these patients is the increase in RAAS as a result of diuresis, renal vasoconstriction, and an accompanying drop in GFR. Although a CVD treatment goal remains to achieve euvolemia (fluid balance), the Acute Decompensated Heart Failure Registry (ADHERE) has noted a higher mortality rate associated with increased diuretic use. Whether the association is truly causal, however, is uncertain at this time.[45-48]

The usual clinician response to patients with HF is to maintain them on a daily diuretic dose even when the patient is euvolemic. When creatinine increases, the most common "reflex" among providers is to decrease ACEI use when, in fact, the creatinine increase may have been a result of overdiuresis. When the patient is overdiuresed, a rise in creatinine may indicate a drop in transglomerular pressure, which indicates a maladaptive response to volume loss and ultimately an

Table 1.4A

Target doses of ACE inhibitors with doses converted to enalapril as the predicate. Doses of 2 FDA-approved angiotensin receptor blockers for heart failure with target doses as used in the clinical trials.

ACE Inhibitor	Starting Dose	Target Dose	Manufacturer's Maximal Dose	Approximate Daily Dose Conversion to Enalapril
Benazepril	5–10 mg qd	20 mg qd	40 mg bid	1:1
Captopril[§,‡]	6.25–12.5 mg tid	50 mg tid	100 mg tid	7.5:1
Enalapril[§,†]	2.5–5 mg bid	10 mg bid	20 mg bid	
Fosinopril[§]	5–10 mg qd	20 mg qd	40 mg qd	1:1
Lisinopril[§,‡]	2.5–5 mg bid	10 mg bid	20 mg bid	1:1
Quinapril[§]	5 mg bid	20 mg bid	40 mg bid	2:1
Ramipril[§,‡]	1.25–2.5 mg bid	5 mg bid	10 mg bid	1:2

All ACE Inhibitors have generic options marketed in the United States. [§]FDA approved for treatment of heart failure. [†]Mortality benefit in large heart failure trial. [‡]Mortality benefit large post-MI or CAD risk factor trial.

ARB*	Starting Dose	Target Dose	Maximal Dose
Candesartan (Atacand®)	4–8 mg daily	32 mg daily	32 mg daily
Valsartan (Diovan®)	20–40 mg bid (80 mg bid if hypersensitive)	160 mg bid	160 mg bid

*Approved for HF by the FDA.

Table 1.4B

Starting and target doses of β blockers with mortality data in heart failure. Both metoprolol succinate (XL) and carvedilol are FDA approved for heart failure.

Agent	Starting Dose	Target Dose <75–85 kg	Target Dose >75–85 kg
Bisoprolol	1.25 mg PO daily	5 mg PO daily	10 mg PO daily
Carvedilol	3.125 mg PO bid	25 mg PO bid	50 mg PO bid
Metoprolol XL	25 mg PO daily* 12.5 mg PO daily[†]	200 mg PO daily	200 mg PO daily

*NYHA class II.

[†]NYHA class III and IV.

increase in renin with further renal vasoconstriction. However, data now show that the rise in creatinine is temporary and that renal function stabilizes after 2 to 3 days.[49-50] The rise in creatinine after administering ACEIs may be related to blood pressure drop in the presence of extensive diuresis. Thus, all possible efforts should be made not to withdraw life-saving therapies (eg, ACEIs).[51]

A recent clinical trial of aldosterone blockade earlier in HF treatment showed significantly positive results for all study end points. The EMPHASIS-HF trial studied eplerenone in patients who had NYHA class II–III HFREF. Findings were positive for improving both mortality and morbidity in these patients.[52] Although eplerenone (aldosterone blockade) is not in the current ACC/AHA Guidelines, it is entirely possible that these findings will be included in the next revision. Careful follow-up of potassium levels is critical when using aldosterone blockade in addition to ACEIs or ARBs.

Devices

In HFREF, the risk of sudden death is a reality even if patients are doing well and have only NYHA class II disease. ICDs are indicated for patients whose EF remains low (<35%) despite being on optimal medication regimens (ie, properly uptitrated), especially β blockers.[53] In one large clinical trial that included both ischemic and nonischemic HF, ICDs were found to be superior to pharmacotherapy with amiodarone.[54] Healthcare providers are well advised to discuss ICDs with their patients so that the latter understand the risks and benefits and can decide whether to accept this intervention. For patients with advanced (class IV) HF, the discussion may include the need to deactivate the ICD in the event that the patient chooses to enroll in hospice care.

In recent years, cardiac resynchronization therapy (CRT), also known as biventricular pacing, has taken its place in the

ACC/AHA Guidelines.[55] CRT may improve ventricular activation when dyssynchrony exists. A left bundle branch block (LBBB) morphology can be indicative of ventricle dyssynchrony. Also, the presence of a wide QRS pattern and an LBBB morphology together serve as a surrogate for dyssynchrony. A QRS interval >120 milliseconds with an LBBB pattern and NYHA class III–IV HF symptoms despite optimal medical therapy are considered indications for CRT to improve patients' functional capacity and quality of life. At least one study has shown that CRT improves survival as well.[56] It should be noted, however, that not all patients benefit from CRT, so carefully selecting only patients with true dyssynchrony is essential. Patients being considered for this therapy should be referred to an HF specialist for consultation.

Lifestyle Counseling: Diet and Physical Activity

Patient education, including lifestyle counseling, has been demonstrated to be effective for many patients with HF.[57-58] The focus of lifestyle counseling generally includes instructions on diet (eg, low-sodium foods and fewer, smaller meals), smoking cessation, and the importance of physical activity. Low-sodium diets are generally recommended for patients with HF, although a recent Cochrane review[59] concluded that evidence was insufficient to determine their relative benefits or drawbacks.

Smoking cessation programs are widespread and have been found to be effective in many groups of patients. Because of the adverse effects of smoking on patients with HF, smoking cessation programs should be offered across sites of care. In fact, smoking cessation is one of the measures in the evidence-based ACC/AHA Guidelines for the treatment of patients with HF.[60]

Despite anecdotal concerns that physical activity for patients with HF might be unsafe, numerous randomized controlled trials (RCTs) have demonstrated that aerobic exercise and physical activity are in fact safe for patients with HF and yield positive outcomes in intervention groups. Benefits include greater exercise capacity, lowered heart rate, reduced inflammatory cytokines, lower all-cause mortality, fewer hospital stays, and improved health status.[61] Although patients with HF may need to adapt their activity level to the physical limits imposed by their disease status, physical activity should be encouraged for all patients with HF. Physical activity for the most impaired patients may consist simply of walking. Resistance training has also found to be safe and effective.[62]

Effective lifestyle counseling should include more than a patient education approach. It should also incorporate elements of "coaching" to encourage lifestyle changes or the use of motivational interviewing techniques to identify patient-identified barriers to beneficial changes.[63] Barriers to lifestyle changes include poor access to healthy foods or to healthy meal preparation, restricted access to safe sites for physical activity, and inadequate insurance coverage for prescription medications. For more on this subject, the reader is referred to an excellent work on motivational interviewing by Emmons et al.[64]

Education and Self-monitoring

Patient education comprises a broad approach to bridging knowledge gaps in patients with HF. It makes use of several approaches, including written materials, audiovisual materials, Internet-based education programs, and increasingly, education through remote telemonitoring systems. The challenge of implementing HF educational programs is that many offer a one-size-fits-all approach rather than one that is tailored to the specific patient's knowledge level and needs. Another obstacle is that few (11%) patient education materials for HF even meet the criteria for health literacy or suitability of content.[65]

Complicating patient education for those with HF are the subtle cognitive changes that accompany the syndrome, known as executive function impairment (EFI). While the etiology of EFI is multifaceted and includes inflammatory causes, hypoxia, and other factors, EFI compromises a person's judgment and decision-making ability regarding self-care and leads to poor recall of information, such as educational materials. Because other comorbid diseases also contribute to EFI, patient educational approaches consisting only of content are less likely to be effective than those that use multifaceted approaches. For example, approaches that include cognitive-behavioral strategies have been found to be more effective than those that include only educational approaches.[66] Self-care and self-monitoring have been studied in a number of RCTs and other studies. They have found that intervention group subjects attained more HF-related knowledge, better self-management (eg, daily weights, sodium restriction, medication management, symptom surveillance), and improved outcomes when engaged by clinicians in self-care activities.[67-68]

AHA has developed a scientific statement that summarizes the current state of the science for promoting self-care in HF. For HF self-care, the organization makes a series of distinct recommendations:

1. Take medications on time and regularly.
2. Self-monitor for symptoms and signs of worsening HF.
3. Keep to a diet of 2 gm to 4 gm of sodium.
4. Limit alcohol intake.
5. Lose weight if excessive body mass index (BMI) (> 40 kg/m^2).

6. Perform routine activity in stable, compensated HF patients.
7. Smoking cessation.[69]

Nutritional Supplementation

All patients with HF should follow the heart-healthy diet recommendations of the national organizations (eg, AHA). A wide variety of patient education materials have been developed and should be offered to patients, tailored to their preferred language and culture.

Researchers have speculated that either the pathophysiological effects of HF or the effects of standard medication for treatment result in depletion of some nutrients. As a result, they have investigated whether nutritional supplements may be beneficial in HF. Several nutritional supplements are recommended for persons with HF, although research evidence on their efficacy has been mixed, and few studies specific to patients with HF have been conducted.[70] Also, in some cases, the mechanisms of action of purported beneficial effects of supplementation have not been established.

NUTRITIONAL ASSESSMENT IN HEART FAILURE PATIENTS

Caveat: Providers are encouraged to carefully consider the most recent research and to examine the possibility of drug–drug interactions, including those of vitamins and minerals with prescription medications, before prescribing or recommending nutritional supplements.

HF patients and their family and friends often seek out advice and prescriptions for nutritional supplements. It is difficult to determine which supplements have any benefit at all, and do no harm. More importantly, one must determine whether they cause any problems (eg, malabsorption of prescription medicines). Another drawback to supplements is that they can be costly, so patients may be better served by spending their money on substances that have proven benefits. For example, eating fish may be preferable to taking expensive fish oil capsules. The following sections touch on supplements for which there is evidence of benefit.

Fish oil

A component of fish oil, n-3 polyunsaturated fatty acids (n-3 PUFA), has been found to have a small but beneficial effect on patients with NYHA class II–IV HF. This finding was based on one randomized, placebo-controlled trial in patients with chronic heart failure (the GISSI-HF trial), which examined the effect on mortality and cardiovascular hospitalizations.[71]

Co-enzyme Q10

Evidence from a systematic review of 11 studies shows that co-enzyme Q10 exerts a small but beneficial effect on EF and cardiac output in patients with heart failure.[72]

Vitamins and minerals

In a comprehensive review, Alsafwah and colleagues found evidence in support of supplementation with magnesium, calcium, vitamin D, thiamin, zinc, and selenium. They pointed out that much of the research that had been done used only one study supplement at a time rather than testing out multivitamin supplement formulations, and the authors touted a role for minerals and micronutrients in certain HF patients.[73]

Rehabilitation Options

Currently, most health insurance programs have limited coverage for cardiac rehabilitation for patients with HF. For example, the Medicare program will not pay for cardiac rehabilitation for patients with HF who are in skilled nursing facilities. This payment gap is a symptom of the fragmentation of the U.S. healthcare system. As a result, providers who want rehabilitation for their patients with HF need to order specific services that are offered in the most appropriate setting. For example, patients with HF who are homebound (require considerable and taxing effort to leave the home) may benefit from home healthcare services for nursing (medication instruction, patient education, and disease surveillance) and physical therapy (for a prescribed exercise program based on disease status and the patient's capacity for exercise). The prescribed exercise program order should include intensity, frequency, duration, and progression.[74] For patients with HF who are able to leave their home, outpatient physical therapy may be beneficial in combination with an educational program designed to promote evidence-based self-management of HF.

The HF-ACTION (Heart Failure: A Controlled Trial Investigating Outcomes of Exercise Training) trial randomized 2,331 patients with NYHA class II–IV systolic HF to an exercise program or a control group. Although the reduction in the primary end point of all-cause mortality or hospitalization was modest, the exercise therapy was found to be safe.[75] In addition, the exercise group had a significant increase in health status, including quality of life.[76]

SPECIAL CONSIDERATIONS FOR SUBGROUPS

Older Adults

The population with HF aged 85 years and older, because of the challenges associated with advanced age and the likelihood of comorbid diseases, merits special consideration for treatment. Pharmacological treatment requires special caution because these patients are likely to have coexisting renal and hepatic disease, which decreases drug clearance.[77-78] Nonetheless, retrospective studies that looked at trials involving this older patient population have shown not only the same benefit of HF drugs but perhaps better results than in the younger age-groups.[79] Therefore, medical therapy should not be withheld solely due to age. Instead, careful upward titration is indicated, recognizing that treatment may be complex because of multiple comorbidities.

Patient and family preferences as to treatment will be specific and may range from aggressive treatment (implantation of devices) to palliative care or hospice. Advance care planning discussions require collaboration among multiple providers. Primary care providers, geriatricians, cardiologists, nurses, and social workers should collaborate to determine patient and family preferences and to provide expertise as the decisions are made. Decisions about advance care planning are more dynamic than they first appear, and one-time discussions are generally inadequate. As the disease progresses, patients and families may change their preferences over time.[80-81]

Women

Women are twice as likely to develop HFpEF as men. Hypothetical sex-related physiological differences in cardiovascular functioning, complicated by age and comorbid disease, are both associated with higher prevalence of HFpEF.[82] Morbidity and mortality for those with HFpEF is similar to those with HFREF,[83] with similar rates of rehospitalization at 60 to 90 days, emergency room visits, and hospital length of stay for HF treatment.[84] Pharmacological treatment for HFpEF has not been established. Various RCTs found minimal or no beneficial effect from a variety of drug classes used to treat HFREF.[85,86] Thus, because evidence-based treatment options are limited, clinical judgment must be used to establish treatment algorithms.

Patients with Diabetes

The obesity epidemic has greatly increased the incidence of diabetes, which is independently associated with the development of CVD in general, and HF in particular.[87] Tight glycemic control reduces microvascular complications and may also reduce macrovascular ones.[88] However, universal pharmacological treatment protocols regarding tight control of blood glucose have not been established.[89] The benefits of weight loss apply to everyone, but especially to those with diabetes. The American Diabetes Association (ADA) recommendations for treating diabetes with blood pressure control, addressing dyslipidemia, antiplatelet therapy, and smoking cessation are also relevant to HF management.[90]

Persons at End of Life

Persons with NYHA class III and IV HF experience significant disease burden—exceeding that of patients with solid tumors. Unlike a cancer diagnosis, however, predicting end-of-life status is challenging for patients with HF, a substantial proportion of whom will succumb to sudden cardiac death. Despite these challenges, end-of-life and advance care planning discussions are recommended during the course of treatment. These can address patient and family preferences regarding the aggressiveness of care and technology to be provided.

A consensus statement has been developed based on the proceedings of a conference (funded by the Agency for Healthcare Research and Quality and the Robert Wood Johnson Foundation) about the current state of palliative and supportive care in advanced HF.[91] Experts came to the following conclusions:

1. Although supportive care should be integrated throughout treatment of patients with advanced HF, data are needed to understand how to best decrease physical

and psychosocial burdens of advanced HF and to meet patient and family needs;

2. Prognostication in advanced HF is difficult and data are needed to understand which patients will benefit from which interventions and how best to counsel patients with advanced HF;
3. Research is needed to identify which interventions improve quality of life and best achieve the outcomes desired by patients and family members;
4. Care should be coordinated between sites of care, and barriers to evidence-based practice must be addressed programmatically; and
5. More research is needed to identify the content and technique of communicating prognosis and treatment options with patients with advanced HF; physicians caring for patients with advanced HF must develop skills to better integrate the patient's preferences into the goals of care.

In addition, the authors provided extensive clinical recommendations for the care of persons with advanced HF.[92]

It is therefore important to involve end-of-life or palliation teams earlier in the care of HF patients. This is true particularly if symptoms are not being controlled with current evidence-based care and the patient may not be eligible for more advanced therapies, such as mechanical devices.

FOLLOW-UP PROCEDURES

When patients with HF are discharged from the hospital, a variety of interventions have been found effective for reducing subsequent rehospitalizations. These include transitional care programs, prompt physician follow-up after the initial hospital stay, telemonitoring, and coordination of care programs, usually nurse-led but multidisciplinary in nature.[93-95]

Transitional care programs are being tested as part of demonstration projects for the Patient Protection and Affordable Care Act of 2010 ("healthcare reform"), which is due to be implemented fully in 2014. Boult and colleagues provided a synthesis of meta-analyses and systematic reviews that demonstrates the positive impact of many of the comprehensive care models on outcomes for patients with HF.[96] Thus, the implementation and integration of components of these models are likely to be effective in improving patient outcomes, including by reducing rehospitalization rates.

Physician Follow-up

Prompt physician follow-up after a hospital stay has been identified as one strategy to reduce the likelihood of rehospitalization. Jencks and colleagues, in a seminal work, determined that approximately half of 11,855,702 Medicare patients (all diagnoses, based on 2002–2003 claims) did not see a physician between hospital discharge and rehospitalization.[97] Because of the importance of adjusting (ie, up-titrating) medications in patients with HF, and because of the need to involve the primary care physician in follow-up care, experts recommend that prompt physician visits be scheduled following a hospital stay.[98] Alternatively, if physician visits are not readily scheduled, follow-up with other healthcare providers (eg, nurses or pharmacists) can be effective. Protocols that would allow these other health professionals to up-titrate medical therapy are not only possible to develop but can be safely deployed. These health professionals are often adept at patient education and are highly valuable members of the treatment team. Ways to further develop their roles are found in Section II of this book: "Multidisciplinary Collaborative Care Model for Patients with Heart Failure."

Telemedicine

Telemonitoring takes many forms for patients with HF. These range from text messaging on cell phones (eg, using mHealth, a mobile healthcare technology provider) to live videoconferencing between patients and nurses and/or physicians. Although the effectiveness of telemonitoring for improving patient outcomes has been mixed, as studied in systematic reviews and meta-analyses, this has not stopped the growth of telemonitoring by providers of all types.[99-102]

Research into care coordination programs has provided mixed results on efficacy and cost-effectiveness. Despite the mixed results, many hospitals and healthcare systems have implemented or are testing various approaches to improve discharge planning and the transition from hospital to home by providing care coordination.[103]

Section II

Multidisciplinary Collaborative Care Model for Patients with Heart Failure

Because the number of individuals living with HF is projected to grow, and this growth will have a large impact on the healthcare system, the benefits of interdisciplinary teams have been a focus of healthcare reform. National registries have been developed for HF patient care, including "Get with the Guidelines–HF" from the American Heart Association, OPTIMIZE-HF, and others.[104-106] All these efforts focus on optimizing HF patient care by using a team-based approach. The team members may change from site to site, but most often, they include physicians (hospitalists, intensivists, cardiologists, internists, and primary care physicians); advanced practice providers (nurse practitioners [NPs], clinical nurse specialists, and physician assistants); registered nurses; dietitians; social workers; and pharmacists. (Although recognition of the importance of physical therapists is increasing, they are less involved than are the other disciplines.) Members of a cardiac rehabilitation team are also considered team members. Multidisciplinary teams function as rounding teams in a variety of settings: acute care, specialized acute care units, outpatient clinics, medical homes, provider offices, community clinics, and home-based care. This section gives an overview of the contributions that various team members (nurses, pharmacists, nutritionists, and physicians) make to HF patient care and concludes with two case studies.

CHAPTER 2

The Nurse's Role in Caring for Patients with Heart Failure

Nancy Altice, DNP, RN, CCNS, ACNS-BC

LICENSED INDEPENDENT PROVIDERS

The advanced practice registered nurse (APRN) may serve as a licensed independent provider (LIP) on a multidisciplinary HF treatment team. In this role, the APRN provides nursing and medical management based on established evidence-based guidelines, such as the Heart Failure Society of America 2010 guidelines and the American College of Cardiology/American Heart Association (ACC/AHA) Guidelines in Chapter 1.[107-108] Because the population served consists primarily of HF patients, the nurse develops specialty expertise in diagnosing and managing HF patients across all stages of the disease and works with physicians from multiple specialties (eg, internal medicine, cardiology).

Identifying and managing comorbid conditions is also essential for improving outcomes in the HF population. Common comorbid conditions include coronary artery disease (CAD), hypertension, diabetes, sleep disordered breathing (eg, sleep apnea), depression, renal insufficiency, and chronic obstructive pulmonary disease (COPD). Executive function impairment (EFI) and cognitive impairment also complicate the management of HF. Therefore, when assessing and treating HF, healthcare providers must take into consideration the impact of these other conditions. For example, managing the medications of

Heart Failure: Strategies to Improve Outcomes © 2013 Joseph S. Alpert, Lynne T. Braun, Barbara J. Fletcher, Gerald Fletcher, Editors-in-chief. Cardiotext Publishing, ISBN: 978-1-935395-50-8.

patients with HF and coexisting renal dysfunction may require one to modify the selection of medications. In some models, the multidisciplinary team manages comorbid conditions directly, but often, other specialists or generalists are needed, with whom the team needs to develop effective partnerships. Mental health problems can coexist in patients with HF, including moderate to severe depression or dementia, so these patients may benefit from the involvement of geropsychiatric specialists. Patients with HF and diabetes may benefit from the involvement of an endocrinologist and a diabetes educator.

Registered nurses (RNs) who are not APRNs can also be team members in many locations. Their license precludes them from prescribing medications or ordering laboratory tests, but their assessment and patient management skills may be critical to team performance and attaining optimal patient outcomes.

PATIENT AND FAMILY ASSESSMENT

Each member of the team completes an assessment based on his or her specific discipline. The nursing assessment is usually comprehensive, including a thorough review of the patient's symptoms, a physical assessment, review of available laboratory and diagnostic information, medication review and reconciliation, and functional and psychosocial screening. A variety of tools may be used to identify comorbid conditions such as depression, cognitive impairment, and sleep apnea. Examples of screening tools for depression include the Patient Health Questionnaire-2 (PHQ2) or the Center for Epidemiologic Studies–Depression (CES-D), both of which are in the public domain. Cognitive impairment screening tools may include the Mini Mental Status Exam (MMSE) or the MiniCog Assessment.

Several aspects of the assessment deserve intense scrutiny: the patient's reported symptoms and their correlation to the other components of the physical assessment and diagnostic findings. It is important to determine whether the patient has identified and correctly interpreted changes that may have been occurring over a period of days or weeks before the encounter. Taking time to explore the patient's interpretation of various symptoms and the resultant decision making is essential for developing interventions that will enhance the patient's self-management skills.

A learning needs assessment should be completed to identify the patient's learning preferences, learning barriers, and priority learning needs. Because family members and other caregivers often assist the patient, it is helpful to determine the preferences for all key learners.[109] In addition, addressing health literacy needs can improve patient education results.

Based on the needs identified during the assessment, the nurse is often the team member who identifies and coordinates referrals to other providers. In some teams, the process automatically includes all members of the team. However, if this is not feasible, the nurse (perhaps in tandem with the physician) screens for needs that can best be met by other disciplines and coordinates a schedule for including these providers.

TEAM COORDINATOR

As the member of the team who may see the patient and family most frequently, the nurse often serves as coordinator and communicator. The advantage of an interdisciplinary approach is that the patient receives care from a variety of experts who consider the patient's individual needs, functional status, comorbid conditions, and social circumstances in order to provide tailored, more effective interventions and education. When multiple providers interact with the patient and family, good communication among team members is essential to ensure that comprehensive instructions are understood by the patient and that potentially contradictory information has been clarified. For example, a physical therapist may instruct the patient to increase activity while the physician, pharmacist, or nurse may have instructed the patient to rest throughout the day and elevate legs for a period of time after taking a diuretic. Thus, without a coordinated approach, the patient may feel frustrated by seemingly conflicting instructions. The nurse, as central coordinator, is in an ideal position to serve as interpreter for the patient, painting the "big picture" of how the various recommendations fit together into a comprehensive plan of care. Follow-up communications to the team may consist of either informal, nonstructured conversations or more structured written communications or team conferences. The nurse is often the member of the team who coordinates these efforts.

PATIENT EDUCATION PROCESSES AND MATERIALS

The team should become familiar with resources available for patient education. A variety of formats, including audiovisual options, should be included to assist learners, including those who prefer this medium as well as those who have reading deficits. Written materials should be evaluated for reading level and other characteristics that aid learning, such as pictures and graphic formatting that simplify and support the messages. Only 12% of adults have proficient health literacy according to the National Assessment of Adult Literacy.[110] This means that more than 8 out of 10 adults may lack the skills needed to manage their health. Myriad resources are available to guide the development of effective written materials. Because many HF patients are older adults, it is also important to consider font size and print color that are easy to read for patients with impaired vision. Materials need to be accessible in multiple languages and include content that is culturally appealing.[111-112]

Materials used by the team should be evaluated for their effectiveness. All members of the team can contribute to this process, but often, nurses have received more formal training on patient education and may be better able to mentor the team in choosing or developing effective education materials and programs. Despite utilizing appropriate materials and evidence-based education approaches, learning may still be limited. Regardless of the patient's perceived health literacy, numerous factors can interfere with learning, including stress, EFI, sleep deprivation, and medication effects. Using the "teach back" method, in which patients are asked to explain in their own words what they have learned and what actions they will take, is an effective way to evaluate whether patients have learned the material. The next step is to evaluate whether the lesson has resulted in the desired outcome of improved self-care.

SELF-CARE

Teaching that results in self-care is a key component of multidisciplinary care. In self-care, the patient actively participates in managing his or her disease or condition. Self-care involves maintenance, management, and evaluation.[113] *Self-care maintenance* refers to active participation and adherence to a healthy lifestyle and prescribed treatments. *Self-care management* entails effective problem solving in the face of changing signs and symptoms, followed by *self-evaluation* of effectiveness. Nurse researchers and clinicians have developed much of the expertise that exists in this realm.[114]

The nurse on the team should be well versed in this literature and able to guide the rest of the team toward effective approaches. As an illustration, a patient may be able to report his or her signs and symptoms yet fail to do so. At this point, it is important to evaluate what the patient understands and how he or she has interpreted reporting instructions. For example, the patient may be able to state that he will report increased shortness of breath. However, the patient may find that limiting activities and sleeping in a recliner relieves this symptom for a period of time and so may believe this symptom is of no significance to report. Another patient may state that a weight gain of 2 to 4 pounds should be reported but gain 10 to 12 pounds before reporting it. On further investigation, the nurse discovers that a patient has been losing weight recently but did not consider this 10- to 12-lb weight loss to be significant until the previous baseline weight had been surpassed. Patients also vary in their somatic awareness. For instance, patients who have been observed by family members to be breathing with significant difficulty may deny being short of breath. Situations such as these require additional education and individualized coaching to help the patient to recognize causes and effects, learn to recognize bodily cues (not deny or minimize them), and effectively solve problems.

GROUP SUPPORT

Cardiac Rehabilitation

No matter how well nurses educate, counsel, and medically treat patients individually, added value can come from interactions with other HF patients. The nurse's role may be to refer the patient to an existing cardiac rehabilitation program or support group. Cardiac rehabilitation provides the additional benefit of monitored exercise, which can reassure patients that they can safely exercise by learning to follow individualized guidelines for activities and paying attention to bodily signals that warn of overexertion. Patients in this setting usually develop connections with other participants and share concerns, empathy, helpful advice, and emotional support. In a support group, the education provided stimulates questions, elicits practical tips from patients who are living with HF, and may increase motivation to actively self-manage the condition.

Shared Medical Appointments

Another option is to consider is the shared medical appointment. In such a clinic, patients are scheduled for a longer than usual medical appointment. The appointment consists of multiple private interviews and assessments with the healthcare team, followed by a group education and support session with team members. These sessions involve nutritionists, psychologists, social workers, and nurses.

TRANSITIONS

Patients require coordinated transition when being readmitted to acute care facilities. In some models, the APRN (or a heart failure nurse coordinator [RN] from the outpatient clinic), follows patients who are readmitted to the hospital to either provide ongoing management or to assist with effective transitions among providers and settings.[115] Depending on the HF services available, other models can contribute to effective transitions. If outpatient care is provided by a variety of healthcare practitioners in multiple locations other than an HF clinic, it can be very helpful to have a nurse in the hospital play the role of clinical nurse specialist, HF coordinator, or case manager. That nurse then thoroughly reviews the needs of the HF patient and coordinates a well-communicated plan to all providers, arranging for the necessary referrals and appointments following hospital discharge. This person can determine whether the patient is eligible for home health care, telehealth monitoring, hospice, cardiac rehabilitation, or even skilled nursing facility placement.

The alarming rehospitalization rates in the United States are of major focus among healthcare payers, so the need for transitional care approaches is pressing. Transitions are a time of risk for patients because, often, they involve changes in medication, functional status, cognitive functioning, and emotional response. This juncture is ideal for reevaluating the medication regimen with the input of pharmacist and physician to identify simpler medication approaches that will facilitate adherence. Patients may need to absorb new information and effectively change their self-care routine to avoid another readmission to the hospital. A number of projects are under way that are testing various approaches to transitional care for patients with HF as part of national healthcare reform efforts.

FOLLOW-UP APPOINTMENTS AND PATIENT-INITIATED COMMUNICATIONS

After being discharged from the hospital after an acute exacerbation of HF, the patient should have contact with a medical professional within 7 days. This time frame is advised by the American College of Cardiology Hospital to Home (H2H) program (http://H2Hquality.org). This time frame can decrease the risk of hospital readmission in several ways: by identifying any misconceptions the patient has about new instructions, determining whether the patient is following the prescribed medication regimen, noting side effects of treatment or new symptoms that are not being adequately treated, and making sure that the patient knows the correct action to take when symptoms or other problems arise. Because current hospital practice has patients being seen by a hospitalist or intensivist rather than their primary care provider, this follow-up appointment is critical. This initial postdischarge follow-up can be provided by a nurse practitioner, clinical nurse specialist, physician assistant, or physician. Depending on the services and facilities available, it may be difficult to obtain an appointment within 7 days, so creative strategies may be needed. For example, the Carilion HF Clinic at the Carilion Roanoke Memorial Hospital offers a one-time transitional follow-up appointment with non–HF clinic physicians to HF patients whose cardiologist or primary care provider is unable to meet with them in the 7-day time frame.

Patients often wait until symptoms are severe before making contact, so it is imperative to clearly discuss expectations with the patient and to evaluate and document the patient's understanding. Discuss the patient's presenting symptoms and their severity at the time of the hospital admission. For example, if the patient presented with extreme dyspnea but had significant weight gain or edema that was not previously reported to the provider, this should be discussed. The patient needs to understand the importance of these signs and how to avoid worsening HF by treating these signs earlier. Patients often delay a consultation because they already have an appointment and don't recognize the need to reschedule when their condition changes.

Every HF patient needs to know when and how to contact the healthcare provider. The nurse can coach the patient on how to handle roadblocks, such as a receptionist who offers an appointment in 3 weeks when the patient is having an acute change of condition. Patients can be taught key information to provide that will make their needs clearer. For example, reporting weight trends, edema, changes in urine output, and degree of dyspnea can give a clearer picture. The patient needs to know how to make contact when the provider's office is closed. Knowing when to call emergency medical services is also essential.

PALLIATIVE/END-OF-LIFE CARE

Palliative care focuses on symptom control. Interdisciplinary teams working with chronic disease patient populations usually take a holistic approach that addresses quality of life and involves patients and families in decisions. These teams are often skilled at helping the patient clarify his or her treatment goals and communicating these to the family, who may have opposing goals. They give patients options for care that range from palliative care to more aggressive interventions, such as implanted ventricular assist devices (VADs) or a heart transplant. All members of the team help to identify the patient's perspective on these approaches. For example, the nurse often has ongoing communication with the patient and may be one of the first to identify indicators that the patient desires a less medically aggressive approach. Palliative care teams can enhance care throughout the stages of HF, and standard medical guidelines can be followed simultaneously with palliative care approaches. During the transition to palliative care, the pharmacist can be helpful in identifying medications that may no longer be necessary or whose dose can be reduced. Also, the nurse can serve as the patient's advocate for identifying alternative approaches in a timely manner and keeping the team involved in developing a comprehensive plan of care.

COORDINATION WITH POST–ACUTE CARE SETTINGS

Nurses can motivate the HF care team to strive for the highest quality possible for each patient. All patients followed up by the team who have unplanned readmissions to the hospital should be reviewed thoroughly to determine whether the causes were avoidable. In this way, the team might identify recurring problems in processes or barriers that could be eliminated to improve care for other patients.

The nurse plays a key role in educating other nurses and healthcare professionals who may be involved in HF care. For example, in the Carilion HF Clinic, we found that many patients who went to skilled nursing facilities were being readmitted within 30 days with significant weight gain and volume overload. After consulting with the nursing administrators at several nursing home facilities, we discovered that some of these facilities could offer a no-added-salt diet but not a true low-sodium diet. The patients were still receiving a variety of high-sodium foods even though salt packets were withheld from their trays. Furthermore, weight gain was not being interpreted as problematic because, in general, the bigger concern at these nursing homes was nutritional deficiency and weight loss. One of their key quality indicators was weight maintenance, so subtle weight gain did not concern them. In this case, a staff education program on HF was developed and presented in these facilities.

Nurse-led HF clinics have been shown to improve patient outcomes,[116] and evidence shows that they also are cost-effective.[117-118] There also is evidence demonstrating that transitional care models that extensively involve nurses are effective at improving patient outcomes during the high-risk period of hospital discharge.[119]

CONCLUSION

Interdisciplinary HF teams can be developed around the unique characteristics of available members and facilities where they will practice. The nurse is an essential member of the team, whose role will usually evolve over time. As expertise grows, and members of the team learn from each other, more effective and efficient ways to collaborate and coordinate care are sure to follow.

CHAPTER 3

The Pharmacist's Role in Caring for Patients with Heart Failure

Angela Cheng-Lai, PharmD, BCPS

Studies have shown that cardiovascular medications reduce morbidity, mortality, and hospitalizations in patients with HF.[120-123] Unfortunately, approximately 50% of patients with chronic diseases do not take their medications as directed, and such nonadherence can lead to cardiac decompensation and subsequent hospitalization in patients with HF.[124-126] Therefore, to improve medication compliance and subsequent clinical outcomes, factors leading to medication nonadherence, such as lack of patient knowledge, lack of follow-up appointments, undesirable side effects, and high drug costs, must be addressed.

IMPACT OF PHARMACIST INTERVENTIONS ON HEART FAILURE PATIENTS

Because of their expertise in drug therapy, pharmacists are particularly well suited to provide the necessary medication education to patients to improve medication adherence.[127] According to an RCT by investigators for the Prevention Trial of the Studies of Left Ventricular Dysfunction (SOLVD), in a 9-month period, a significant improvement in medication compliance was observed in 106 patients who received medication counseling by a pharmacist belonging to an interdisciplinary team, compared with 164 patients who did not receive extensive pharmacist counseling. Medication adherence was 78.8% and

Heart Failure: Strategies to Improve Outcomes © 2013 Joseph S. Alpert, Lynne T. Braun, Barbara J. Fletcher, Gerald Fletcher, Editors-in-chief. Cardiotext Publishing, ISBN: 978-1-935395-50-8.

67.9% in the pharmacist-intervention and usual care groups, respectively (95% CI, 5.0% to 16.7%).[128] In addition, emergency department visits and hospital admissions were 19.4% less frequent (incidence rate ratio, 0.82 [CI, 0.73 to 0.93]) and annual direct healthcare costs lower by $2,960 per patient (CI, –$7,603 to $1,338) in the pharmacist-intervention group.[129]

As demonstrated in the SOLVD Prevention Trial, pharmacists can play an important role in a multidisciplinary team and help improve outcomes in patients with HF. However, there is less evidence to support the role of pharmacist as an individual healthcare provider. A meta-analysis of 12 RCTs involving 2,060 patients was conducted to clarify the role of pharmacists—both as a member of a multidisciplinary team (in pharmacist collaborative care) and as the key driver of interventions (in pharmacist-directed care).[130] Researchers found that pharmacist collaborative care was associated with significant reductions in the rate of all-cause hospitalizations (OR, 0.71; 95% CI, 0.54 to 0.94) and hospitalizations due to HF (OR, 0.69; 95% CI, 0.51 to 0.94) and a nonsignificant reduction in mortality (OR, 0.84; 95% CI, 0.61 to 1.15). Of note, pharmacist collaborative care led to greater reductions in the rate of hospitalizations due to HF (OR, 0.42; 95% CI, 0.24 to 0.74) than did pharmacist-directed care (OR, 0.89; 95% CI, 0.68 to 1.17). Thus, including a pharmacist in the care of patients with HF—particularly within a multidisciplinary team—is likely to benefit patients and should be strongly encouraged.

HEART FAILURE PATIENT CARE INITIATIVE: THE PHARMACIST'S ROLE

As an example of the role of the pharmacist, we describe a program being developed at Montefiore Einstein Medical Center in the Bronx, New York, a center of excellence that has been at the forefront of healthcare initiatives and strives to provide the best care for all patients. Because HF patients have high mortality and hospitalization rates, it is important to optimize the care of these patients in order to reduce their rates of morbidity and mortality. For this reason, a multidisciplinary care team is being assembled to improve the care and outcomes of HF patients at this medical center. Encouraged by positive results from published studies, multidisciplinary teams in HF clinics will include pharmacists. They will play several crucial roles: educating patients about their medication regimens (giving them written information when appropriate), resolving medication-related problems (eg, drug interactions; adverse effects; compliance problems; use of unnecessary, inappropriate, or duplicate medicines; inappropriate dosage; and out-of-date medicines), and assessing the patient's need for compliance aids.[131] In collaboration with a cardiologist, pharmacists will adjust dosages of ACEIs, β blockers, and diuretics in order to optimize the effects of these medications. Pharmacists may accomplish the above tasks during the initial patient counseling session and in subsequent telephone follow-up interviews.

INITIAL PATIENT EDUCATION SESSION CONDUCTED BY PHARMACISTS

In an effort to improve the care and health outcomes of HF patients, AHA has launched a nationwide campaign to address CVD. This campaign offers healthcare providers comprehensive tools to guide the care of heart failure patients. HF tools: http://www.heart.org/HEARTORG/HealthcareResearch/GetWithTheGuidelinesHFStroke/GetWithTheGuidelines-HeartFailureHomePage/Heart-Failure-Clinical-Tools-Library_UCM_305817_Article.jsp

According to AHA, at least 60 minutes of patient education in single or divided sections are needed in order to ensure that the patient understands what actions must be taken after hospital discharge. Nine domains should be covered during the 60 minutes:

1. How to recognize escalating symptoms and concretely plan how to respond to particular symptoms
2. Recommendations for activity and exercise
3. Indications, use, and need for adherence to each medication prescribed at discharge
4. Importance of monitoring one's weight daily
5. Ways to modify risk factors for HF progression (eg, smoking cessation, managing weight and blood pressure)
6. Specific diet recommendations (eg, for an individualized low-sodium diet or to cut down on alcohol intake)
7. Follow-up appointments
8. Discharge instructions
9. End of life

Pharmacists are most well versed in domain number 3. Written educational materials, such as the Heart Failure Patient Education Booklet (prepared by the HF team at Montefiore Einstein Medical Center), which cover many of these domains, should be given to the patient as an educational resource. Other healthcare professionals (eg, physicians, nurses, dietitians) from the multidisciplinary team are involved in addressing the above domains and reinforcing patient education. At the conclusion of the patient education session, the pharmacist will document in the patient's medical record domains that were addressed.

FOLLOW-UP TELEPHONE INTERVIEWS

A follow-up phone call can help to assess not only the patient's health status, but also whether the patient truly understands the facts. Patients need to comprehend the causes of HF, their disease prognosis, medication therapy, dietary restrictions, allowable activities, and the importance of self-care, and recognize the signs and symptoms of worsening HF. The AHA provides a telephone follow-up form that can be utilized for patient interviews (www.myamericanheart.org). According to AHA, it is important to assess the following areas of knowledge during a follow-up phone call:

- Does the patient know the signs and symptoms of HF and what to do if he or she experiences any signs or symptoms?
- Is the patient currently taking medications that were prescribed at discharge?
- Does the patient understand why taking these medications is important?
- If the medicine supply runs low, does the patient have access to an adequate backup supply?
- If the patient is not taking prescribed medications, what is the rationale?
- Can the patient manage a flexible diuretic regimen to treat worsening signs and symptoms of volume overload?
- Does the patient have any questions about diet, activity, medications, or other subjects?
- Has the patient completed a scheduled follow-up appointment?
- Does the patient understand the importance of the follow-up visit?

Because many of these follow-up questions are medication related, pharmacists may be the ideal healthcare providers to conduct these interviews. Alternatively, the interviews may be conducted by other members of the multidisciplinary team (eg, nurses) with a pharmacist giving input and consulting on medication-related questions and issues. Information gathered from these interviews will be recorded on the AHA follow-up phone call form. This information will help to assess any further patient needs and, in turn, help to optimize care and health outcomes.

SUMMARY

Pharmacists can be an essential part of a multidisciplinary team caring for patients with HF. To test this approach, in 2012, pharmacists joined the multidisciplinary HF treatment team at Montefiore in counseling patients with HF. With the support of a multidisciplinary team, pharmacists conduct initial patient education sessions and telephone follow-up interviews. It is expected that this collaborative effort will improve the care and outcome of our HF patients.

CHAPTER 4

The Nutritionist's Role in Caring for Patients with Heart Failure

Miriam Pappo, MS, RD, CDN

Risk factors for worsening HF include high blood pressure, high blood cholesterol, being overweight or obese, diabetes, smoking, lack of physical activity, and depression and other emotional health difficulties. Because lifestyle—especially nutrition—is a key component of HF prevention and management, registered dietitians (RDs) are integral to a strong multidisciplinary HF team.

ROLE OF THE CARDIAC DIETITIAN

Cardiac dietitians treat people with heart disease and other cardiac-related illnesses. They specialize in providing nutritional services that aim to prevent heart disease from worsening and promote heart health and wellness through preventive nutrition counseling and medical nutrition therapy (MNT). The following are key areas of a dietitian's responsibility for maintaining the nutritional health of cardiovascular patients and reducing CVD risk:

- Education and counseling on healthy eating habits
- Weight management
- Diabetes management
- Smoking cessation
- Sports and exercise nutrition
- Meal preparation and cooking demonstrations
- Complementary (alternative) nutrition approaches to CVD

Heart Failure: Strategies to Improve Outcomes © 2013 Joseph S. Alpert, Lynne T. Braun, Barbara J. Fletcher, Gerald Fletcher, Editors-in-chief. Cardiotext Publishing, ISBN: 978-1-935395-50-8.

- Body-fat testing
- Improvement in lipid values
- Reduction in blood pressure
- Protecting bone health
- Postsurgical wound healing

The goals of nutritional intervention are to improve biochemical markers of risk, such as serum insulin, into a more desirable range, and to lower the patient's weight, serum lipids, blood pressure, and blood sugar by modifying their diet. These interventions are particularly relevant for patients with HF because of the impact that diet has on the development of HF symptoms. Also, because HF is the culmination of other types of heart disease, MNT for managing cardiac disease is crucial. Finally, because patients with HF frequently have other comorbid diseases (eg, diabetes), the cardiac dietitian can play a key role in developing a nutritional plan that addresses multiple chronic diseases.

NUTRITION EDUCATION

The dietitian's nutrition education responsibilities include one-on-one nutrition assessment and consultation. The dietitian also helps to design and implement nutrition classes for outpatient cardiac rehabilitation patients, including those with HF. Dietitians consult with physicians and nurses and interpret laboratory values, assess dietary patterns, and analyze the nutrient composition of foods using computer software. Through these techniques, the dietitian devises an individualized care plan, sets goals, and makes recommendations. He or she monitors the patient's progress with carefully kept records and re-education when needed.

A diet and education program is designed to encourage compliance with dietary restrictions and modifications while addressing factors such as food allergies, likes and dislikes, cultural preferences, and each individual's accessibility to certain foods. The dietitian or nutritionist teaches clients ways to change their eating habits and clarifies and identifies obstacles to diet modification. The dietitian uses motivational interviewing and other counseling skills to help the patient to achieve a more self-directed, healthy lifestyle.

RESEARCH FINDINGS SUPPORTING OUTCOMES AND EFFECTIVENESS

Studies have found that ongoing nutritional counseling achieves greater outcomes than one-time instruction.[132] Ongoing guidance to patients, and their family and caretakers, allows them to move from theory to the practical incorporation of new habits into their daily life. Questions arise in day-to-day life that can be answered when a dietitian is on the case. Real-life scenarios, such as making sounder choices at a variety of restaurants, holiday eating, special events, and navigating the supermarket aisles, help motivated patients to make gradual yet sustained dietary modifications.

Patients in cardiac rehabilitation programs have experienced greater weight loss when a registered dietitian is on their team. In addition, scores on nutrition knowledge tests increased and resulted in patients reporting making healthier food choices.[133] Delahanty and colleagues reported in their study of patients with high cholesterol that those assigned to a registered dietitian for consultation, as well as MNT, achieved and sustained an 8% decrease in total dietary fat intake (from 32% to 24%) and a 4% decrease in saturated fat intake (from 11% to 7%). These improvements were statistically significant at both 3 and 6 months following MNT.[133]

A study by Timlin et al. demonstrated that, after receiving nutrition education, patients' dietary choices when dining out improved, as did their self-confidence in adhering to a lipid-lowering diet. Patients indicated that, after attending nutrition education classes, they were most confident about which foods to purchase and eat, were better able to decrease dietary fat and cholesterol, and were able to remain on a healthy diet by themselves.[135] This finding concurs with results from the Delahanty study, which concluded that MNT provided by a registered dietitian is a worthwhile investment of resources. They found that MNT given by a dietitian results in significantly higher patient satisfaction levels about understanding lifestyle changes, eating habits, and the role of cholesterol in CVD. In addition, patients counseled by dietitians in this study improved their ability to manage cholesterol levels and eating habits compared with patients who received MNT from physicians and other healthcare professionals.[136]

Scant research exists on the specific contributions that MNT makes to the treatment of patients with HF. Systematic reviews and meta-analyses have identified the inclusion of dietitians in the multidisciplinary team,[137,138] but no recent studies have evaluated the individual contributions that cardiac dietitians make to improving HF patient outcomes. Despite this lack of evidence, the complexity of care and the importance of nutritional intake by patients with HF strongly recommend that dietitians be involved as part of the multidisciplinary team.

SUMMARY

Working in a cardiac care setting requires active listening skills. Critical thinking and solid problem-solving ability are prerequisites. Analytic and deductive reasoning are needed to interpret a combination of cardiac risk factors, such as obesity, diabetes, high blood pressure, and hyperlipidemia, which often present at the same time. Maintaining currency in and applying new research findings are paramount ways to ensure the excellence of the team. It is understandable that the American public is confused about food selections and therefore prone to making misinformed decisions. Individuals need help sifting through the current popular fad diets and lifestyle recommendations that abound in the mass media. The cardiac dietitian has the professional resources available to set both the team and HF patients straight.

CHAPTER 5

The Physician's Role in Caring for Patients with Heart Failure

Snehal Patel, MD

Traditional physician training and clinical practice emphasize treating the individual patient. Therefore, it comes as no surprise that physicians have been slow to embrace the HF clinic—a disease management program that emphasizes the treatment of populations and diffuses the physician-centric approach to healthcare delivery. Nonetheless, the rationale of the HF clinic is clear: Large gaps exist in translating the results of evidence-based therapies to patients with chronic conditions such as HF. The multidisciplinary approach of the HF clinic seeks to remedy this situation. By providing extended patient education, motivation, and support for adherence to the prescribed initiated therapies, including lifestyle changes, the HF clinic complements the traditional role of the physician. Ultimately, in order for the HF clinic to succeed, the physician must embrace this multidisciplinary approach.

Accumulating outcomes data and cost-effectiveness studies provide a compelling mandate that these programs must be adopted. In a retrospective study, Akosah and colleagues demonstrated that, after index hospitalization for HF, patients followed up by their usual physicians had a mortality rate 2.4 times higher than patients followed up at an HF clinic.[139] A prospective trial from the Netherlands randomized patients to either an HF clinic or usual care provided by individual cardiologists at two academic medical centers. Despite the high standard of care in the control group, researchers found a significant decrease in the

Heart Failure: Strategies to Improve Outcomes © 2013 Joseph S. Alpert, Lynne T. Braun, Barbara J. Fletcher, Gerald Fletcher, Editors-in-chief. Cardiotext Publishing, ISBN: 978-1-935395-50-8.

composite end point of HF hospitalizations and all-cause mortality over 1 year of follow-up. In addition, significant differences were noted in favor of the HF clinic group in left ventricular ejection fraction (LVEF) improvement, quality of life, NYHA class, and healthcare costs.[140] Numerous other studies conducted within the United States and internationally have confirmed these benefits of the HF clinic.

Based on these compelling findings, it is clear that the HF clinic will redefine the healthcare delivery model, as it utilizes a multidisciplinary, collaborative approach. The physician's role in this model has been drastically altered. No longer are physicians the sole proprietors of patient care; rather, this responsibility has now been spread to other members of a team that includes nutritionists, social workers, pharmacists, nurses, nurse practitioners, and physician assistants. Despite this diffusion of responsibilities, a successful program will require the physician to take a leadership role in a variety of areas. Table 5.1 outlines the important roles of the physician in the HF clinic.

Table 5.1
Physicians' Role in the Heart Failure Clinic

Pharmacotherapy and device protocols	• Create care pathways that optimize medical therapy, as detailed in the most recent HF practice guidelines. • Maintain algorithms that ensure that ICDs and biventricular pacing are offered to eligible candidates. • Update protocols based on the most recent literature, which may not yet have been incorporated into published guidelines.
Patient triage within the clinic	• Begin initial patient evaluation upon entry into the clinic. • Assign patients to appropriate clinical care pathways based on diagnosis and level of mental acuity.

Table 5.1 ***continued*** Physicians' Role in the Heart Failure Clinic	
Consultation with advanced practice providers	• Provide medical expertise when advanced practice nurses or physician assistants identify a patient who requires augmented levels of care or deviates from defined care pathways (eg, a patient with ischemic cardiomyopathy who develops new ventricular arrhythmias or unstable angina).
Continuity during transitions of care	• Provide continuity of care during the transition from inpatient to outpatient setting. • Ensure timeliness of follow-up after discharge for acute exacerbations of HF (ie, within 72 hours for complex cases and 7 to 10 days for routine patients).

PHARMACOTHERAPY AND DEVICE PROTOCOLS

The physician is responsible for creating clinical care pathways that delineate algorithms for the initiation and up-titration of appropriate evidence-based medical therapies. These protocols should be based on current HF guidelines but should also periodically be updated to incorporate new findings not yet included in the guidelines. The algorithms should also include contingencies for commonly encountered adverse events, such as symptomatic hypotension and worsening renal function. These algorithms are then utilized by advanced practice providers as a template for patient management.

PATIENT TRIAGE

At the time of patient entry into the clinic, the initial evaluation should be performed by a physician. After the appropriate diagnosis is made and a plan for management is in place, the physician can transition the patient to a clinical care pathway to be followed by an advanced practice provider. This is particularly important for patients with nontraditional cardiomyopathies (eg, amyloid heart disease, hypertrophic cardiomyopathy) or advanced HF that is likely to require heart transplantation, LVAD, or end-of-life management.

CONSULTATION WITH ADVANCED PRACTICE PROVIDERS

The heterogeneity of the HF disease process, coupled with its natural course of progression and high prevalence of comorbidities, suggests that patients followed within the clinic will frequently deviate from the clinical care protocols. In such instances, the physician should be available to provide input and, if necessary, consultation to optimize patient management.

CONTINUITY DURING TRANSITIONS OF CARE

Management of patients with HF takes place on a continuum—from treatment of acute exacerbations in the hospital setting to chronic management in the clinic setting. In many instances, physicians provide the only link between these two settings, and it is therefore their responsibility to maintain appropriate continuity of care. In fact, the literature cites inadequate discharge planning, poor follow-up, noncompliance with medication, and dietary nonadherence as frequent preventable causes of hospital readmissions.[141] The most effective discharge planning occurs when the physician from the HF clinic communicates with the physicians providing care in the hospital setting (eg, hospitalists, intensivists) so that the treatment plans can be continued or appropriately modified.

In conclusion, the HF clinic is a multidisciplinary, collaborative approach to disease management that utilizes a variety of integrated measures to improve patient outcomes, enhance quality of life, and reduce healthcare costs. In this paradigm, the physician is no longer the focal point of healthcare delivery. Although the physicians' role has changed, they will maintain a variety of responsibilities that are no less important. Ultimately, for HF clinics to reach their full potential, physicians must embrace their new calling.

CHAPTER 6

The Social Worker's Role in Caring for Patients with Heart Failure

Xiomara Tolentino, LMSW

Similar to other healthcare professionals, the role of social workers is to improve patient quality of life by evaluating patients' psychosocial environment.[142] By doing this, social workers are ensuring that the patient has a stable environment and support system, which makes patient care easier and potentially more effective.

ROLE OF THE SOCIAL WORKER IN PATIENT DISCHARGE

When patients with HF are discharged from hospitals, social workers facilitate the patients' discharge experience by providing the necessary paperwork, including insurance forms and forms for home healthcare procedures. Social workers also educate HF patients and their loved ones about the patients' condition and helpful ways in which to live with HF once the patient is discharged from the medical facility. For example, education on the expected emotional responses to living with a progressive chronic illness like HF can help patients understand their feelings. Social workers also may evaluate the need for equipment (eg, durable medical equipment like a bedside commode) or other services (eg, home-delivered meals, assistance with bathing from a home health aide) that will support patient independence at the same time as addressing safety.

Heart Failure: Strategies to Improve Outcomes © 2013 Joseph S. Alpert, Lynne T. Braun, Barbara J. Fletcher, Gerald Fletcher, Editors-in-chief. Cardiotext Publishing, ISBN: 978-1-935395-50-8.

LINKING PATIENTS TO OUTSIDE SERVICES

In addition to the transitioning patients into the home setting, social workers make referrals for community-based social service activities and agencies and to community-based resources for any chronic, disabling, and life-threatening diseases such as HF, as well as for physical rehabilitation.[142] Social workers will also inform patients about any government benefits for which they are eligible and arrange transportation methods for HF patients who need to go from medical facilities to their home and vice versa.[143] Social workers make sure to accommodate patients as much as possible by providing support and by maintaining a constant interest in patients' healthcare and overall well-being.

COLLABORATION WITH OTHER MEMBERS OF THE TEAM

Social workers, as members of the multidisciplinary team, communicate their findings to and coordinate care (eg, referrals) with other members of the team via case conferences, clinical documentation, and informal communication. Social workers sometimes are provided details on social and family circumstances about which other members of the healthcare team may not be aware. Therefore, their input and collaboration is particularly important for identifying obstacles that may interfere with medical management (eg, lack of funding for medications). Also, social workers possess expertise on the availability of specialized community resources that are geographically specific (eg, from neighborhood block grants) and changes to social service programs (eg, in eligibility for home-delivered meals because of state funding cuts).[144-145]

SUMMARY

Social workers are important members of the multidisciplinary care team for patients with HF. They play important roles assisting with discharge planning and giving anticipatory guidance on responses to chronic illness. Coordination and collaboration are key components in the effective management of patients with HF, and social workers are trained to link people in need to the right resources.

Section III

Case Studies

Case Study #1

PF is a 59-year-old white male with a history of hypertension for 20 years, complaining of recent dyspnea on exertion. He was seen 1 month ago by his internist for exertional dyspnea, at which time he was diagnosed with HF (with an LVEF of 15%) and treated with digoxin, a loop diuretic, and an ACEI.

His symptoms improved and he was referred to the HF clinic for further evaluation.

Level of activity:
PF admitted to intermittent fatigue and a slight-to-moderate limitation of his normal activities during the past few months.

Physical examination findings:

- BP: 126/84 mm Hg
- HR: 82 bpm
- HEENT (head, eyes, ears, nose, and throat) exam: no JVD present
- Lungs: clear
- Heart: left ventricular S3 was noted
- No ascites or pedal edema

Laboratory data:

- Serum creatinine: 1.4 mg/dL
- Potassium: 4.7 mEq/L
- LVEF: 15%
- Left ventricular end diastolic pressure 250 mL/m^2

Heart Failure: Strategies to Improve Outcomes © 2013 Joseph S. Alpert, Lynne T. Braun, Barbara J. Fletcher, Gerald Fletcher, Editors-in-chief. Cardiotext Publishing, ISBN: 978-1-935395-50-8.

- No history suggestive of angina
- Electrocardiogram showed no evidence of prior MI

He is determined to have NYHA class II HF and is stable on his current medication regimen.

WHAT WOULD YOU DO NOW AND WHY?

Based on their proven morbidity and mortality benefits in large-scale clinical trials, β blockers are recommended for the treatment of patients with HF due to left ventricular systolic dysfunction. They are to be added to standard therapy of diuretics, ACEIs, and (sometimes) digoxin in clinically stable patients.

Based on the findings from MERIT-HF (Metoprolol CR/XL Randomized Intervention Trial in Congestive Heart Failure),[146] metoprolol succinate should be initiated at 25 mg once daily in patients with NYHA class II HF. The dose should then be doubled every 2 weeks to the highest dose level tolerated by the patient, or up to 200 mg. The dose must be individualized and closely monitored during up-titration. Thus, the decision was made to add a β blocker to achieve additional morbidity and mortality benefits. PF was initiated on metoprolol succinate 25 mg once daily and instructed to follow up with the clinic in 4 weeks. PF was also instructed to monitor his weight daily and to call the clinic if weight gain or shortness of breath (SOB) developed.

Three weeks later:

The initial dose of metoprolol succinate was well tolerated, and was doubled to 50 mg once daily. PF reported improvement in his exercise capacity.

One month later:

- Heart rate: 70 bpm
- Blood pressure: 124/82 mm Hg
- No evidence of edema

After 1 month on metoprolol succinate 50 mg once daily, PF continued to do well. The dose was again doubled to 100 mg once daily.

The 2-month follow-up visit was delayed because PF had a scheduled vacation on a cruise. He continued all his medications during the cruise at the current doses but ate fast food and abandoned his low-sodium diet. During the 1-week trip, he gained 8 pounds and noted increased SOB. Upon his return, he requested an urgent appointment to be seen.

PF was determined to be in decompensated HF, and consideration was given to whether he needed hospitalization or could be managed with closely monitored outpatient care. The decision was made to manage him with close outpatient care with a 3-day follow up by the clinic nurse practitioner. The reason for the decompensated HF was not intolerance to β blockade but rather increased sodium intake with resulting fluid retention. Current HF guidelines recommend that if patients experience mild or moderate worsening of HF symptoms, β-blocker treatment should be continued while the patient is stabilized by optimizing diuretic and ACE inhibitor therapies. Abrupt withdrawal of β-blocker therapy can lead to clinical deterioration and should be avoided. The decision was made to increase the dose of the diuretic (with increased potassium replacement) and to maintain PF on his current β-blocker dose.

PF's dose of furosemide was increased to 80 mg daily for 1 week, administered with 20 mEq of potassium chloride. His dose of metoprolol succinate was maintained at 100 mg once daily. The importance of salt restriction was reinforced, and PF was instructed to follow up in the clinic in 3 days and then 2 weeks if his condition had improved. He lost 6 pounds, and his SOB resolved within the 3 days. Two weeks later, upon his return to the clinic, his weight was stable, BP 124/82, heart rate 68 bpm, and no edema.

Two months later:

PF returns to the clinic, reports that his activity level is improving and that he is walking every day. PF is currently euvolemic and clinically stable. Current HF guidelines recommend that β blockers be titrated, as tolerated, to achieve the target dose.[147] The decision was made to increase the β-blocker dose to achieve the maximum morbidity and mortality benefits of β blockade, as demonstrated in clinical trials. The dose of metoprolol succinate was increased to 150 mg once daily, and PF was scheduled to return in 1 month to complete upward titration to the target dose of 200 mg once daily. PF is being followed on a routine basis, generally every 4 months for evaluation of his HF status, with his medication regimen maintained as ordered.

Case Study #2

MR, a 77-year-old African American female, is referred to the HF clinic following a 3-day hospitalization for acute decompensated HF. She has a history of dyspnea on exertion and orthopnea, which led to the hospitalization. She works part-time as a cashier in a local diner, where she eats 2 of her 3 meals every day. Her BMI is 35 and her EF is 22%. She is widowed and lives alone; her two children are in good health but live out of state. The patient reports that her mother was a diabetic and died suddenly in her 60s. The patient was taking metformin 1 gm bid, as prescribed by her primary care provider, but insists "I do not have sugar." She was on no cardiac medications prior to this hospitalization and admitted that she had not seen her primary care provider for more than 2 years. She also asserts, "I do not like taking medication, so get me off of all these medicines!"

She was discharged on the following medications:

- Metformin 1 gm bid
- Furosemide 40 mg bid
- Amlodipine 5 mg qd
- Valsartan 80 mg qd
- Carvedilol 6.25 mg bid

At the first visit with the physician, Mrs. R was prescribed valsartan 80 mg bid, and with the increase in the angiotensin II receptor blocker (ARB), the amlodipine was

Heart Failure: Strategies to Improve Outcomes © 2013 Joseph S. Alpert, Lynne T. Braun, Barbara J. Fletcher, Gerald Fletcher, Editors-in-chief. Cardiotext Publishing, ISBN: 978-1-935395-50-8.

stopped because the patient needed a simpler regimen for compliance. Therefore, most of her medications were taken twice a day.

She was asked to return 2 weeks later. The clinic utilized group appointments, and Mrs. R was identified as an ideal candidate as she has a new medication, a recent hospitalization, and concern about how much she understands self-management of her health conditions. At the first group visit, the nutritionist spent time with the group reviewing the importance of a low-sodium diet, explaining that, even with ideal medication regimens, failure to follow a low-sodium diet inevitably results in exacerbation of HF. Mrs. R is attentive but does not take the printed handouts when she leaves. During her time in the exam room with the NP, she is noted to have slightly elevated BP (146/88) but a normal pulse and no pedal or other edema. Her JVP is normal at 8 cm. The NP up-titrates her β blocker to carvedilol 12.5 bid but keeps the other medications as prescribed. A return visit is scheduled for 2 weeks.

At the next 2-week appointment, Mrs. R does not show up. A phone call by the clinic RN finds that Mrs. R "forgot" the appointment but reports she is doing well. She is asked to come in 2 weeks later. At this group appointment, the NP discusses the importance of physical activity and even walking. Mrs. R openly scoffs at this suggestion and retorts, "Old people should not exercise." She is not willing to consider increasing her physical activity. During her individual appointment, the NP notes that Mrs. R has slight dyspnea on exertion and slight pedal edema. Mrs. R admits to having had a "nice piece" of ham the day before at the diner. The NP increases the furosemide dose to 80 mg bid for 3 days along with a potassium supplement. Upon follow-up, Mrs. R reports her swelling is down and her breathing has improved.

Mrs. R continues with this pattern of missing periodic follow-up visits and expressing reluctance to follow recommended advice for diet and physical activity, although she does take her medications as prescribed. At one of the group visits she attends, the social worker is talking about emotional reactions to having HF and coping strategies, and Mrs. R starts to cry. She is referred to and follows up with the psychiatric NP, who diagnoses her with moderate depressive symptoms and starts her on a selective serotonin reuptake inhibitor. The psychiatric NP explains that the medication will take up to 6 weeks to provide relief and follows up in 6 weeks. At this time, Mrs. R says she is feeling better "in the head" and agrees to continue on the antidepressant.

Two years following her initial contact with the clinic, Mrs. R has an inferior-wall MI, requiring a hospital stay, and she receives a stent. Following this hospitalization, she returns to the group visits but is barely engaged in the conversations and is very quiet when seeing the physician and NPs. Her functional abilities have declined to the point where it takes considerable effort for her to move. Upon referral to the psychiatric NP, Mrs. R discloses that she is tired of living, that her husband and friends are "mostly dead," and that she is tired of all the medications, her physical inability, and the diet restrictions. She is no longer able to work, so she cannot see her work friends and spends most of her time alone in her house, watching TV. The psychiatric NP increases the dose of antidepressants, but this does not work to allay Mrs. R's emotional response.

At the next visit 6 weeks later, Mrs. R meets with both the physician and the NP, who initiate discussions regarding her preferences for treatment in the event that her condition deteriorates. Mrs. R repeats her statement that she is tired of living and that she is "ready to go." The advance care planning discussion with Mrs. R is enlightening to the physician and NP, who did not realize that Mrs. R desired no further aggressive treatment. Several weeks later, Mrs. R has another episode of acute decompensated HF and is hospitalized. She refuses several treatments and is discharged with a palliative care consult. The palliative care team manages her medication regimen by simplifying the doses to balance therapeutic benefit with side effects and provides her with an aide to assist her with personal care. Mrs. R is continued on her other medications and her antidepressants. Within a month, Mrs. R has decided to discontinue her own medications and "eat whatever the hell I want." Because she is cognitively intact, the palliative care team, working with the physician, NP, and psychiatric NP try to convince Mrs. R to resume her medications. She refuses and is referred to Adult Protective Services, who judge her as sufficiently competent to make her own medical decisions. Several weeks later, Mrs. R is found dead in her home, with the coroner ruling that she had a massive MI.

During the debrief, the team discusses whether anything else could have been done for Mrs. R. The team initiated advance care planning discussions when the patient indicated her interest in such, provided psychiatric specialist care to manage the depression, and referred her to palliative care when the time came. The conclusion was that the team offered and supported the patient's decisions, even though they did not necessarily agree with them, and that perhaps the discussions about an advance directive should have occurred earlier.

References

1. Lloyd-Jones D, Adams RJ, Brown TM, Carnethon M, Dai S, De Simone G, et al. Heart disease and stroke statistics—2010 update: a report from the American Heart Association. *Circulation*. 2010;121:e46–e215.
2. Fang J, Mensah GA, Croft JB, Keenan NL. Heart failure-related hospitalization in the U.S., 1979 to 2004. *J Am Coll Cardiol*. 2008;52:428–434.
3. Jencks SF, Williams MV, Coleman EA. Rehospitalizations among patients in the Medicare fee-for-service program. *N Engl J Med*. 2009;360:1418–1428.
4. Lloyd-Jones D, Adams RJ, Brown TM, Carnethon M, Dai S, De Simone G, et al. Heart disease and stroke statistics—2010 update: a report from the American Heart Association. *Circulation*. 2010;121:e46–e215.
5. Haldeman GA, Croft JB, Giles WH, Rashidee A. Hospitalization of patients with heart failure: National Hospital Discharge Survey, 1985 to 1995. *Am Heart J*. 1999;137:352–360.
6. Jencks SF, Williams MV, Coleman EA. Rehospitalizations among patients in the Medicare fee-for-service program. *N Engl J Med*. 2009;360:1418–1428.
7. Adams KF Jr, Fonarow GC, Emerman CL, LeJemtel TH, Costanzo MR, Abraham WT, et al. Characteristics and outcomes of patients hospitalized for heart failure in the United States: rationale, design, and preliminary observations from the first 100,000 cases in the Acute Decompensated Heart Failure National Registry (ADHERE). *Am Heart J*. 2005;149:209–216.
8. O'Connor CM, Whellan DJ, Lee KL, Keteyian SJ, Cooper LS, Ellis SJ, et al. Efficacy and safety of exercise training in patients with chronic heart failure: HF-ACTION randomized controlled trial. *JAMA*. 2009;301:1439–1450.
9. Yusuf S, Pfeffer MA, Swedberg K, Granger CB, Held P, McMurray JJ, et al. Effects of candesartan in patients with chronic heart failure and preserved left-ventricular ejection fraction: the CHARM-Preserved Trial. *Lancet*. 2003;362:777–781.

10. Massie BM, Carson PE, McMurray JJ, Komajda M, McKelvie R, Zile MR, et al. Irbesartan in patients with heart failure and preserved ejection fraction. *N Engl J Med.* 2008;359:2456–2467.
11. The CONSENSUS Trial Study Group. Effects of enalapril on mortality in severe congestive heart failure. Results of the Cooperative North Scandinavian Enalapril Survival Study (CONSENSUS). *N Engl J Med.* 1987;316:1429–1435.
12. O'Connor CM, Whellan DJ, Lee KL, Keteyian SJ, Cooper LS, Ellis SJ, et al. Efficacy and safety of exercise training in patients with chronic heart failure: HF-ACTION randomized controlled trial. *JAMA.* 2009;301:1439–1450.
13. Adams KF Jr, Fonarow GC, Emerman CL, LeJemtel TH, Costanzo MR, Abraham WT, et al. Characteristics and outcomes of patients hospitalized for heart failure in the United States: rationale, design, and preliminary observations from the first 100,000 cases in the Acute Decompensated Heart Failure National Registry (ADHERE). *Am Heart J.* 2005;149:209–216.
14. Yusuf S, Pfeffer MA, Swedberg K, Granger CB, Held P, McMurray JJ, et al. Effects of candesartan in patients with chronic heart failure and preserved left-ventricular ejection fraction: the CHARM-Preserved Trial. *Lancet.* 2003;362:777–781.
15. Massie BM, Carson PE, McMurray JJ, Komajda M, McKelvie R, Zile MR, et al. Irbesartan in patients with heart failure and preserved ejection fraction. *N Engl J Med.* 2008;359:2456–2467.
16. Hunt SA, Abraham WT, Chin MH, Feldman AM, Francis GS, Ganiats TG, et al. 2009 Focused Update Incorporated Into the ACC/AHA 2005 Guidelines for the Diagnosis and Management of Heart Failure in Adults. A Report of the American College of Cardiology Foundation/American Heart Association Task Force on Practice Guidelines: developed in collaboration with the International Society for Heart and Lung Transplantation. *Circulation.* 2009;119:e391–e479.
17. Stewart S, McAlister FA, McMurray JJ. Heart failure management programs reduce readmissions and prolong survival. *Arch Intern Med.* 2005;165:1311–1312.
18. Bentley B, De Jong MJ, Moser DK, Peden AR. Factors related to nonadherence to low sodium diet recommendations in heart failure patients. *Eur J Cardiovasc Nurs.* 2005;4:331–336.
19. Nohria A, Mielniczuk LM, Stevenson LW. Evaluation and monitoring of patients with acute heart failure syndromes. *Am J Cardiol.* 2005;96:32G–40G.
20. Maisel AS. Use of BNP levels in monitoring hospitalized heart failure patients with heart failure. *Heart Fail Rev.* 2003;8:339–344.
21. Januzzi JL Jr, Camargo CA, Anwaruddin S, Baggish AL, Chen AA, Krauser DG, et al. The N-terminal Pro-BNP investigation of

dyspnea in the emergency department (PRIDE) study. *Am J Cardiol.* 2005;95:948–954.

22. Januzzi JL Jr, Rehman SU, Mohammed AA, Bhardwaj A, Barajas L, Barajas J, et al. Use of amino-terminal pro-B-type natriuretic peptide to guide outpatient therapy of patients with chronic left ventricular systolic dysfunction. *J Am Coll Cardiol.* 2011;58:1881–1889.
23. Troughton RW, Richards AM. BNP for clinical monitoring of heart failure. *Heart Fail Clin.* 2006;2:333–343.
24. Jourdain P, Jondeau G, Funck F, Gueffet P, Le Helloco A, Donal E, et al. Plasma brain natriuretic peptide–guided therapy to improve outcome in heart failure: the STARS-BNP Multicenter Study. *J Am Coll Cardiol.* 2007;49:1733–1739.
25. Hunt SA, Abraham WT, Chin MH, Feldman AM, Francis GS, Ganiats TG, et al. 2009 Focused Update Incorporated Into the ACC/AHA 2005 Guidelines for the Diagnosis and Management of Heart Failure in Adults. A Report of the American College of Cardiology Foundation/American Heart Association Task Force on Practice Guidelines: developed in collaboration with the International Society for Heart and Lung Transplantation. *Circulation.* 2009;119:e391–e479.
26. Lindenfeld J, Albert NM, Boehmer JP, Collins SP, Ezekowitz JA, Givertz MM, et al. HFSA 2010 Comprehensive Heart Failure Practice Guideline. *J Card Fail.* 2010;16:e1–e194.
27. The CONSENSUS Trial Study Group. Effects of enalapril on mortality in severe congestive heart failure. Results of the Cooperative North Scandinavian Enalapril Survival Study (CONSENSUS). *N Engl J Med.* 1987;316:1429–1435.
28. The SOLVD Investigators. Effect of enalapril on mortality and the development of heart failure in asymptomatic patients with reduced left ventricular ejection fractions. *N Engl J Med.* 1992;327:685–691.
29. The SOLVD Investigators. Effect of enalapril on survival in patients with reduced left ventricular ejection fractions and congestive heart failure. *N Engl J Med.* 1991;325:293–302.
30. The CONSENSUS Trial Study Group. Effects of enalapril on mortality in severe congestive heart failure. Results of the Cooperative North Scandinavian Enalapril Survival Study (CONSENSUS). *N Engl J Med.* 1987;316:1429–1435.
31. The SOLVD Investigators. Effect of enalapril on survival in patients with reduced left ventricular ejection fractions and congestive heart failure. *N Engl J Med.* 1991;325:293–302.
32. Cohn JN, Tognoni G. A randomized trial of the angiotensin-receptor blocker valsartan in chronic heart failure. *N Engl J Med.* 2001;345:1667–1675.

33. Granger CB, McMurray JJ, Yusuf S, Held P, Michelson EL, Olofsson B et al. Effects of candesartan in patients with chronic heart failure and reduced left-ventricular systolic function intolerant to angiotensin-converting-enzyme inhibitors: the CHARM-Alternative trial. *Lancet.* 2003;362:772–776.
34. Hunt SA, Abraham WT, Chin MH, Feldman AM, Francis GS, Ganiats TG et al. 2009 Focused Update Incorporated Into the ACC/AHA 2005 Guidelines for the Diagnosis and Management of Heart Failure in Adults. A Report of the American College of Cardiology Foundation/American Heart Association Task Force on Practice Guidelines: developed in collaboration with the International Society for Heart and Lung Transplantation. *Circulation.* 2009;119:e391–e479.
35. Waagstein F. Beta blockers in heart failure. *Cardiology.* 1993;82(Suppl 3):13–18.
36. Eichhorn EJ. Restoring function in failing hearts: the effects of beta blockers. *Am J Med.* 1998;104:163–169.
37. Packer M, Fowler MB, Roecker EB, Coats AJ, Katus HA, Krum H, et al. Effect of carvedilol on the morbidity of patients with severe chronic heart failure: results of the Carvedilol Prospective Randomized Cumulative Survival (COPERNICUS) study. *Circulation.* 2002;106:2194–2199.
38. Hjalmarson A, Goldstein S, Fagerberg B, Wedel H, Waagstein F, Kjekshus J et al. Effects of controlled-release metoprolol on total mortality, hospitalizations, and well-being in patients with heart failure: the Metoprolol CR/XL Randomized Intervention Trial in congestive heart failure (MERIT-HF). MERIT-HF Study Group. *JAMA.* 2000;283:1295–1302.
39. The Cardiac Insufficiency Bisoprolol Study II (CIBIS-II): a randomised trial. *Lancet.* 1999;353:9–13.
40. Packer M, Fowler MB, Roecker EB, Coats AJ, Katus HA, Krum H, et al. Effect of carvedilol on the morbidity of patients with severe chronic heart failure: results of the Carvedilol Prospective Randomized Cumulative Survival (COPERNICUS) study. *Circulation.* 2002;106:2194–2199.
41. The Cardiac Insufficiency Bisoprolol Study II (CIBIS-II): a randomised trial. *Lancet.* 1999;353:9–13.
42. Ghali JK, Piña IL, Gottlieb SS, Deedwania PC, Wikstrand JC. Metoprolol CR/XL in female patients with heart failure: analysis of the experience in Metoprolol Extended-Release Randomized Intervention Trial in Heart Failure (MERIT-HF). *Circulation.* 2002;105:1585–1591.
43. Hunt SA, Abraham WT, Chin MH, Feldman AM, Francis GS, Ganiats TG et al. 2009 Focused Update Incorporated Into the ACC/AHA 2005 Guidelines for the Diagnosis and Management of Heart Failure in Adults. A Report of the American College of

Cardiology Foundation/American Heart Association Task Force on Practice Guidelines: developed in collaboration with the International Society for Heart and Lung Transplantation. *Circulation.* 2009;119:e391–e479.

44. Lindenfeld J, Albert NM, Boehmer JP, Collins SP, Ezekowitz JA, Givertz MM, et al. HFSA 2010 Comprehensive Heart Failure Practice Guideline. *J Card Fail.* 2010;16:e1–e194.

45. Kohler GI, Bode-Boger SM, Busse R, Hoopmann M, Welte T, Boger RH. Drug-drug interactions in medical patients: effects of in-hospital treatment and relation to multiple drug use. *Int J Clin Pharmacol Ther.* 2000;38:504–513.

46. Zaidenstein R, Eyal S, Efrati S, Akivison L, Michowitz MK, Nagornov V, et al. Adverse drug events in hospitalized patients treated with cardiovascular drugs and anticoagulants. *Pharmacoepidemiol Drug Saf.* 2002;11:235–238.

47. Peacock WF, Costanzo MR, De Marco T, Lopatin M, Wynne J, Mills RM, et al. Impact of intravenous loop diuretics on outcomes of patients hospitalized with acute decompensated heart failure: insights from the ADHERE registry. *Cardiology.* 2009;113:12–19.

48. Hasselblad V, Gattis SW, Shah MR, Lokhnygina Y, O'Connor CM, Califf RM, et al. Relation between dose of loop diuretics and outcomes in a heart failure population: results of the ESCAPE trial. *Eur J Heart Fail.* 2007;9:1064–1069.

49. Braunstein JB, Anderson GF, Gerstenblith G, Weller W, Niefeld M, Herbert R, et al. Noncardiac comorbidity increases preventable hospitalizations and mortality among Medicare beneficiaries with chronic heart failure. *J Am Coll Cardiol.* 2003;42:1226–1233.

50. Bairey Merz CN, Johnson BD, Sharaf BL, Bittner V, Berga SL, Braunstein GD, et al. Hypoestrogenemia of hypothalamic origin and coronary artery disease in premenopausal women: a report from the NHLBI-sponsored WISE study. *J Am Coll Cardiol.* 2003;41:413–419.

51. Ruggenenti P, Remuzzi G. Worsening kidney function in decompensated heart failure: Treat the heart, don't mind the kidney. *Eur Heart J.* 2011;32:2476–2478.

52. Zannad F, McMurray JJ, Krum H, van Veldhuisen DJ, Swedberg K, Shi H, et al. Eplerenone in patients with systolic heart failure and mild symptoms. *N Engl J Med.* 2011;364:11–21.

53. Hunt SA, Abraham WT, Chin MH, Feldman AM, Francis GS, Ganiats TG et al. 2009 Focused Update Incorporated Into the ACC/AHA 2005 Guidelines for the Diagnosis and Management of Heart Failure in Adults. A Report of the American College of Cardiology Foundation/American Heart Association Task Force on Practice Guidelines: developed in collaboration with the International Society for Heart and Lung Transplantation. *Circulation.* 2009;119:e391–e479.

54. Bardy GH, Lee KL, Mark DB, Poole JE, Packer DL, Boineau R, et al. Amiodarone or an implantable cardioverter-defibrillator for congestive heart failure. *N Engl J Med.* 2005;352:225–237.
55. Hunt SA, Abraham WT, Chin MH, Feldman AM, Francis GS, Ganiats TG, et al. 2009 Focused Update Incorporated Into the ACC/AHA 2005 Guidelines for the Diagnosis and Management of Heart Failure in Adults. A Report of the American College of Cardiology Foundation/American Heart Association Task Force on Practice Guidelines: developed in collaboration with the International Society for Heart and Lung Transplantation. *Circulation.* 2009;119:e391–e479.
56. Bristow MR, Saxon LA, Boehmer J, Krueger S, Kass DA, De Marco T, et al. Cardiac-resynchronization therapy with or without an implantable defibrillator in advanced chronic heart failure. *N Engl J Med.* 2004;350:2140–2150.
57. Arcand JA, Brazel S, Joliffe C, Choleva M, Berkoff F, Allard JP, et al. Education by a dietitian in patients with heart failure results in improved adherence with a sodium-restricted diet: a randomized trial. *Am Heart J.* 2005;150:716.
58. Fonarow GC. Strategies to improve the use of evidence-based heart failure therapies. *Rev Cardiovasc Med.* 2005;6(Suppl 2):S32–S42.
59. Taylor RS, Ashton KE, Moxham T, Hooper L, Ebrahim S. Reduced dietary salt for the prevention of cardiovascular disease. *Cochrane Database Syst Rev.* 2011;CD009217.
60. Hunt SA, Abraham WT, Chin MH, Feldman AM, Francis GS, Ganiats TG et al. 2009 Focused Update Incorporated Into the ACC/AHA 2005 Guidelines for the Diagnosis and Management of Heart Failure in Adults. A Report of the American College of Cardiology Foundation/American Heart Association Task Force on Practice Guidelines: developed in collaboration with the International Society for Heart and Lung Transplantation. *Circulation.* 2009;119:e391–e479.
61. Downing J, Balady GJ. The role of exercise training in heart failure. *J Am Coll Cardiol.* 2011;58:561–569.
62. Piña IL. Cardiac rehabilitation in heart failure: a brief review and recommendations. *Curr Cardiol Rep.* 2010;12:223–229.
63. Miller WR, Rose GS. Toward a theory of motivational interviewing. *Am Psychol.* 2009;64:527–537.
64. Emmons KM, Rollnick S. Motivational interviewing in health care settings. Opportunities and limitations. *Am J Prev Med.* 2001;20:68–74.
65. Taylor-Clarke K, Henry-Okafor Q, Murphy C, Keyes M, Rothman R, Churchwell A, et al. Assessment of commonly available education materials in heart failure clinics. *J Cardiovasc Nurs.* 2011;27:485–494.

66. Barnason S, Zimmerman L, Young L. An integrative review of interventions promoting self-care of patients with heart failure. *J Clin Nurs.* 2012;21:448–475.
67. Moser DK, Dickson V, Jaarsma T, Lee C, Stromberg A, Riegel B. Role of self-care in the patient with heart failure. *Curr Cardiol Rep.* 2012;14:265–275.
68. Riegel B, Lee CS, Dickson VV. Self care in patients with chronic heart failure. *Nat Rev Cardiol.* 2011;8:644–654.
69. Riegel B, Moser DK, Anker SD, Appel LJ, Dunbar SB, Grady KL, et al. State of the science: promoting self-care in persons with heart failure: a scientific statement from the American Heart Association. *Circulation.* 2009;120:1141–1163.
70. Lee JH, Jarreau T, Prasad A, Lavie C, O'Keefe J, Ventura H. *Congest Heart Fail.* Jul-Aug 2011;17(4):199-203.
71. Tavazzi L, Maggioni AP, Marchioli R, Barlera S, Franzosi MG, Latini R et al. Effect of n-3 polyunsaturated fatty acids in patients with chronic heart failure (the GISSI-HF trial): a randomised, double-blind, placebo-controlled trial. *Lancet.* 2008;372:1223–1230.
72. Sander S, Coleman CI, Patel AA, Kluger J, White CM. The impact of coenzyme Q10 on systolic function in patients with chronic heart failure. *J Card Fail.* 2006;12:464–472.
73. Alsafwah S, Laguardia SP, Arroyo M, Dockery BK, Bhattacharya SK, Ahokas RA, et al. Congestive heart failure is a systemic illness: a role for minerals and micronutrients. *Clin Med Res.* 2007;5:238–243.
74. Piña IL. Cardiac rehabilitation in heart failure: a brief review and recommendations. *Curr Cardiol Rep.* 2010;12:223–229.
75. O'Connor CM, Whellan DJ, Lee KL, Keteyian SJ, Cooper LS, Ellis SJ, et al. Efficacy and safety of exercise training in patients with chronic heart failure: HF-ACTION randomized controlled trial. *JAMA.* 2009;301:1439–1450.
76. Flynn KE, Piña IL, Whellan DJ, Lin L, Blumenthal JA, Ellis SJ, et al. Effects of exercise training on health status in patients with chronic heart failure: HF-ACTION randomized controlled trial. *JAMA.* 2009;301:1451–1459.
77. Piña IL, O'Connor C. BNP-guided therapy for heart failure. *JAMA.* 2009;301:432–434.
78. Jourdain P, Jondeau G, Funck F, Gueffet P, Le Helloco A, Donal E, et al. Plasma brain natriuretic peptide–guided therapy to improve outcome in heart failure: the STARS-BNP Multicenter Study. *J Am Coll Cardiol.* 2007;49:1733–1739.
79. Deedwania PC, Gottlieb S, Ghali JK, Waagstein F, Wikstrand JC. Efficacy, safety and tolerability of beta-adrenergic blockade with metoprolol CR/XL in elderly patients with heart failure. *Eur Heart J.* 2004;25:1300–1309.

80. Waterworth S, Gott M. Decision making among older people with advanced heart failure as they transition to dependency and death. *Curr Opin Support Palliat Care.* 2010;4:238–242.
81. Stuart B. Palliative care and hospice in advanced heart failure. *J Palliat Med.* 2007;10:210–228.
82. Scantlebury DC, Borlaug BA. Why are women more likely than men to develop heart failure with preserved ejection fraction? *Curr Opin Cardiol.* 2011;26:562–568.
83. Tsutsui H, Tsuchihashi-Makaya M, Kinugawa S. Clinical characteristics and outcomes of heart failure with preserved ejection fraction: lessons from epidemiological studies. *J Cardiol.* 2010;55:13–22.
84. Fonarow GC, Stough WG, Abraham WT, Albert NM, Gheorghiade M, Greenberg BH, et al. Characteristics, treatments, and outcomes of patients with preserved systolic function hospitalized for heart failure: a report from the OPTIMIZE-HF Registry. *J Am Coll Cardiol.* 2007;50:768–777.
85. *Ibid.*
86. Massie BM, Carson PE, McMurray JJ, Komajda M, McKelvie R, Zile MR, et al. Irbesartan in patients with heart failure and preserved ejection fraction. *N Engl J Med.* 2008;359:2456–2467.
87. Plutzky J. Macrovascular effects and safety issues of therapies for type 2 diabetes. *Am J Cardiol.* 2011;108:25B–32B.
88. *Ibid.*
89. Weiss IA, Valiquette G, Schwarcz MD. Impact of glycemic treatment choices on cardiovascular complications in type 2 diabetes. *Cardiol Rev.* 2009;17:165–175.
90. Executive summary: standards of medical care in diabetes—2010. *Diabetes Care.* 2010;33(Suppl 1):S4–S10.
91. Goodlin SJ, Hauptman PJ, Arnold R, Grady K, Hershberger RE, Kutner J et al. Consensus statement: Palliative and supportive care in advanced heart failure. *J Card Fail.* 2004;10:200–209.
92. *Ibid.*
93. Naylor MD, Bowles KH, Brooten D. Patient problems and advanced practice nurse interventions during transitional care. *Public Health Nurs.* 2000;17:94–102.
94. Naylor MD. Transitional care for older adults: a cost-effective model. *LDI Issue Brief.* 2004;9:1–4.
95. Jencks SF, Williams MV, Coleman EA. Rehospitalizations among patients in the Medicare fee-for-service program. *N Engl J Med.* 2009;360:1418–1428.
96. Boult C, Green AF, Boult LB, Pacala JT, Snyder C, Leff B. Successful models of comprehensive care for older adults with chronic conditions: evidence for the Institute of Medicine's "retooling for an aging America" report. *J Am Geriatr Soc.* 2009;57:2328–2337.

97. Jencks SF, Williams MV, Coleman EA. Rehospitalizations among patients in the Medicare fee-for-service program. *N Engl J Med.* 2009;360:1418–1428.

98. Hernandez AF, Greiner MA, Fonarow GC, Hammill BG, Heidenreich PA, Yancy CW, et al. Relationship between early physician follow-up and 30-day readmission among Medicare beneficiaries hospitalized for heart failure. *JAMA.* 2010;303:1716–1722.

99. Clarke M, Shah A, Sharma U. Systematic review of studies on telemonitoring of patients with congestive heart failure: a meta-analysis. *J Telemed Telecare.* 2011;17:7–14.

100. Inglis SC, Clark RA, McAlister FA, Ball J, Lewinter C, Cullington D, et al. Structured telephone support or telemonitoring programmes for patients with chronic heart failure. *Cochrane Database Syst Rev.* 2010;CD007228.

101. Polisena J, Tran K, Cimon K, Hutton B, McGill S, Palmer K, et al. Home telemonitoring for congestive heart failure: a systematic review and meta-analysis. *J Telemed Telecare.* 2010;16:68–76.

102. Chaudhry SI, Mattera JA, Curtis JP, Spertus JA, Herrin J, Lin Z, et al. Telemonitoring in patients with heart failure. *N Engl J Med.* 2010;363:2301–2309.

103. Peikes D, Chen A, Schore J, Brown R. Effects of care coordination on hospitalization, quality of care, and health care expenditures among Medicare beneficiaries: 15 randomized trials. *JAMA.* 2009;301:603–618.

104. Fonarow GC, Abraham WT, Albert NM, Gattis SW, Gheorghiade M, Greenberg BH, et al. Influence of a performance-improvement initiative on quality of care for patients hospitalized with heart failure: results of the Organized Program to Initiate Lifesaving Treatment in Hospitalized Patients With Heart Failure (OPTIMIZE-HF). *Arch Intern Med.* 2007;167:1493–1502.

105. *Ibid.*

106. Hong Y, LaBresh KA. Overview of the American Heart Association "Get With the Guidelines" programs: coronary heart disease, stroke, and heart failure. *Crit Pathw Cardiol.* 2006;5:179–186.

107. Hunt SA, Abraham WT, Chin MH, Feldman AM, Francis GS, Ganiats TG, et al. 2009 Focused Update Incorporated Into the ACC/AHA 2005 Guidelines for the Diagnosis and Management of Heart Failure in Adults. A Report of the American College of Cardiology Foundation/American Heart Association Task Force on Practice Guidelines: developed in collaboration with the International Society for Heart and Lung Transplantation. *Circulation.* 2009;119:e391–e479.

108. Lindenfeld J, Albert NM, Boehmer JP, Collins SP, Ezekowitz JA, Givertz MM, et al. HFSA 2010 Comprehensive Heart Failure Practice Guideline. *J Card Fail.* 2010;16:e1–e194.

109. Boyde M, Tuckett A, Peters R, Thompson DR, Turner C, Stewart S. Learning style and learning needs of heart failure patients (The Need2Know-HF patient study). *Eur J Cardiovasc Nurs.* 2009;8:316–322.

110. Wilkins F, Bozik K, Bennett K. The impact of patient education and psychosocial supports on return to normalcy 36 months post-kidney transplant. *Clin Transplant.* 2003;17(Suppl 9):78–80.

111. Ridpath J, Greene S. PS1-63: PRISM Online Training: a free, customized, effective plain language tutorial for researchers. *Clin Med Res.* 2012;10:169.

112. Hill-Briggs F, Schumann KP, Dike O. Five-step methodology for evaluation and adaptation of print patient health information to meet the < 5th grade readability criterion. *Med Care.* 2012;50:294–301.

113. Lindenfeld J, Albert NM, Boehmer JP, Collins SP, Ezekowitz JA, Givertz MM, et al. HFSA 2010 Comprehensive Heart Failure Practice Guideline. *J Card Fail.* 2010;16:e1–e194.

114. Richard AA, Shea K. Delineation of self-care and associated concepts. *J Nurs Scholarsh.* 2011;43:255–264.

115. McCauley KM, Bixby MB, Naylor MD. Advanced practice nurse strategies to improve outcomes and reduce cost in elders with heart failure. *Dis Manag.* 2006;9:302–310.

116. Phillips CO, Singa RM, Rubin HR, Jaarsma T. Complexity of program and clinical outcomes of heart failure disease management incorporating specialist nurse-led heart failure clinics. A meta-regression analysis. *Eur J Heart Fail.* 2005;7:333–341.

117. Hebert PL, Sisk JE, Wang JJ, Tuzzio L, Casabianca JM, Chassin MR, et al. Cost-effectiveness of nurse-led disease management for heart failure in an ethnically diverse urban community. *Ann Intern Med.* 2008;149:540–548.

118. Turner DA, Paul S, Stone MA, Juarez-Garcia A, Squire I, Khunti K. Cost-effectiveness of a disease management programme for secondary prevention of coronary heart disease and heart failure in primary care. *Heart.* 2008;94:1601–1606.

119. McCauley KM, Bixby MB, Naylor MD. Advanced practice nurse strategies to improve outcomes and reduce cost in elders with heart failure. *Dis Manag.* 2006;9:302–310.

120. The SOLVD Investigators. Effect of enalapril on survival in patients with reduced left ventricular ejection fractions and congestive heart failure. *N Engl J Med.* 1991;325:293–302.

121. McMurray J, Ostergren J, Pfeffer M, Swedberg K, Granger C, Yusuf S, et al. Clinical features and contemporary management of patients with low and preserved ejection fraction heart failure: baseline characteristics of patients in the Candesartan in Heart failure-Assessment of Reduction in Mortality and morbidity (CHARM) programme. *Eur J Heart Fail.* 2003;5:261–270.

122. Granger CB, McMurray JJ, Yusuf S, Held P, Michelson EL, Olofsson B, et al. Effects of candesartan in patients with chronic heart failure and reduced left-ventricular systolic function intolerant to angiotensin-converting-enzyme inhibitors: the CHARM-Alternative trial. *Lancet.* 2003;362:772–776.
123. Pitt B, Zannad F, Remme WJ, Cody R, Castaigne A, Perez A, et al. The effect of spironolactone on morbidity and mortality in patients with severe heart failure. Randomized Aldactone Evaluation Study Investigators. *N Engl J Med.* 1999;341:709–717.
124. The SOLVD Investigators. Effect of enalapril on survival in patients with reduced left ventricular ejection fractions and congestive heart failure. *N Engl J Med.* 1991;325:293–302.
125. Ghali JK, Krause-Steinrauf HJ, Adams KF, Khan SS, Rosenberg YD, Yancy CW, et al. Gender differences in advanced heart failure: insights from the BEST study. *J Am Coll Cardiol.* 2003;42:2128–2134.
126. Vinson JM, Rich MW, Sperry JC, Shah AS, McNamara T. Early readmission of elderly patients with congestive heart failure. *J Am Geriatr Soc.* 1990;38:1290–1295.
127. Santschi V, Chiolero A, Burnand B, Colosimo AL, Paradis G. Impact of pharmacist care in the management of cardiovascular disease risk factors: a systematic review and meta-analysis of randomized trials. *Arch Intern Med.* 2011;171:1441–1453.
128. The SOLVD Investigators. Effect of enalapril on survival in patients with reduced left ventricular ejection fractions and congestive heart failure. *N Engl J Med.* 1991;325:293–302.
129. *Ibid.*
130. Koshman SL, Charrois TL, Simpson SH, McAlister FA, Tsuyuki RT. Pharmacist care of patients with heart failure: a systematic review of randomized trials. *Arch Intern Med.* 2008;168:687–694.
131. Kalisch LM, Roughead EE, Gilbert AL. Improving heart failure outcomes with pharmacist-physician collaboration: How close are we? *Future Cardiol.* 2010;6:255–268.
132. Bowerman S, Bellman M, Saltsman P, Garvey D, Pimstone K, Skootsky S, et al. Implementation of a primary care physician network obesity management program. *Obes Res.* 2001;9(Suppl 4): 321S–325S.
133. *Ibid.*
134. Delahanty LM, Sonnenberg LM, Hayden D, Nathan DM. Clinical and cost outcomes of medical nutrition therapy for hypercholesterolemia: a controlled trial. *J Am Diet Assoc.* 2001;101:1012–1023.
135. Timlin MT, Shores KV, Reicks M. Behavior change outcomes in an outpatient cardiac rehabilitation program. *J Am Diet Assoc.* 2002;102:664–671.
136. Delahanty LM, Sonnenberg LM, Hayden D, Nathan DM. Clinical and cost outcomes of medical nutrition therapy for hypercholesterolemia: a controlled trial. *J Am Diet Assoc.* 2001;101:1012–1023.

137. Holland R, Battersby J, Harvey I, Lenaghan E, Smith J, Hay L. Systematic review of multidisciplinary interventions in heart failure. *Heart.* 2005;91:899–906.

138. Jaarsma T. Health care professionals in a heart failure team. *Eur J Heart Fail.* 2005;7:343–349.

139. Akosah KO, Schaper AM, Haus LM, Mathiason MA, Barnhart SI, McHugh VL. Improving outcomes in heart failure in the community: long-term survival benefit of a disease-management program. *Chest.* 2005;127:2042–2048.

140. de la Porte PW, Lok DJ, van Veldhuisen DJ, van Wijngaarden J, Cornel JH, Zuithoff NP, et al. Added value of a physician-and-nurse-directed heart failure clinic: results from the Deventer–Alkmaar heart failure study. *Heart.* 2007;93:819–825.

141. Vinson JM, Rich MW, Sperry JC, Shah AS, McNamara T. Early readmission of elderly patients with congestive heart failure. *J Am Geriatr Soc.* 1990;38:1290–1295.

142. DuBois BL, Miley KK. *Social Work: An Empowering Profession.* New York: Prentice Hall; 2010.

143. Popple P, Leighninger L. *Social Work, Social Welfare and American Society.* 8th ed. New York: Prentice Hall; 2010.

144. Hepworth DH. *Direct Social Work Practice: Theory and Skills.* New York: Brooks Cole; 2009.

145. Moralese AT, Sheafor BW. *Social Work: A Profession of Many Faces.* New York: Prentice Hall; 2011.

146. Hjalmarson A, Goldstein S, Fagerberg B, Wedel H, Waagstein F, Kjekshus J, et al. Effects of controlled-release metoprolol on total mortality, hospitalizations, and well-being in patients with heart failure: the Metoprolol CR/XL Randomized Intervention Trial in congestive heart failure (MERIT-HF). MERIT-HF Study Group. *JAMA.* 2000;283:1295–1302.

147. Hunt SA, Abraham WT, Chin MH, Feldman AM, Francis GS, Ganiats TG et al. 2009 Focused Update Incorporated Into the ACC/AHA 2005 Guidelines for the Diagnosis and Management of Heart Failure in Adults. A Report of the American College of Cardiology Foundation/American Heart Association Task Force on Practice Guidelines: Developed in collaboration with the International Society for Heart and Lung Transplantation. *Circulation.* 2009;119:e391–e479.

Index

Page numbers followed by *f*, *t*, refer to figures, tables